# GET A BETTER NIGHT'S SLEEP

**Ian Oswald,** an eminent professor of psychiatry, runs the sleep research laboratory at Edinburgh University in Scotland. The President of the European Sleep Research Society, Professor Oswald has had numerous papers on sleep published in scientific and medical journals, and two of his books about sleep have been translated into several languages.

**Kirstine Adam,** a biochemist, brings her research interest in food and bodily metabolism to the field of sleep research. A member of the Association for the Psychophysiological Study of Sleep, she has written articles on dietary habits and sleep, sleep as a restorative process, and sleeping pills.

The authors, who are married, share a special love of plants, gardens and the Scottish hills, as well as good food and interesting wines.

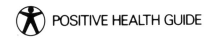 POSITIVE HEALTH GUIDE

# GET A BETTER NIGHT'S SLEEP

Ian Oswald
MD, FRCPsych, DSc

**and**

Kirstine Adam
PhD

Arco Publishing, Inc.
New York

Published 1983 by Arco Publishing, Inc.
215 Park Avenue South, New York, N.Y. 10003

First published in the United Kingdom in 1983
by Martin Dunitz Ltd, London

**Library of Congress Cataloging in Publication Data**
Oswald, Ian.
    Get a better night's sleep.
    (Positive health guide)
    Includes index.
    1. Insomnia.    2. Sleep disorders.    I. Adam, Kirstine.
II. Title.    III. Series.
RC548.078        616.8'49        82–4060
                                AACR2
ISBN 0–668–05335–6 (hardcover)


Phototypeset in Garamond by Input Typesetting Ltd, London

Printed in Singapore by Koon Wah Printing Pte Ltd

# CONTENTS

# INTRODUCTION

We all sleep, but many people wish they could sleep better. Indeed, most of us have experienced difficulties in sleeping at some time in our lives. We know, for example, that around 15 per cent of patients attending their family doctor complain of insomnia, and that in middle-age, and later, at least one woman in four habitually takes either prescribed medicines or over-the-counter preparations in the hope of improving sleep. Many use bedtime food drinks, and even more drink alcohol, with the same expectation. Problems with sleeping, then, are a very common, and sometimes distressing experience.

Everyday anxieties are often to blame. An accident to your child, the news that a loved one is ill or pressures of work or business can leave any of us tense and awake with unhappy preoccupations in the night. The very fact of being awake is to many a source of worry; needless worry, as we shall be explaining. A few broken nights, though unpleasant, are not going to have any serious consequences, and in time the original worry will become reduced and better sleep will return. Some of you will, we are sure, reply that you do not feel refreshed by sleep, irrespective of any current problem in life; or that you are prevented from getting a good night's sleep by other things such as noise, shift-work, wakeful babies, breathing difficulties, and so forth; or that as you have become older you find it more difficult to sleep. For you, and for any with a more general desire to learn about sleep, we hope this book will be of value.

We write having between us some thirty-five years of special experience of research into all aspects of sleep, and an awareness of the most common anxieties and questions people have about sleep. At Edinburgh we have been fortunate in having excellent laboratories for studying the sleep of hundreds of volunteers by monitoring their electrical brain waves, but have learned just as much by what people tell us of their own sleep. Numerical figures, precise measurement, and statistical comparisons are the tools of research; plain experience of what people feel about their sleep, and a willingness to listen, add a necessary extra.

Research brings about a little advance in knowledge here, another little advance there, it settles one small question after another. By gradual increase of knowledge on a broad front, and not by dramatic breakthroughs, we come to new understandings about the nature of sleep, which in the long run, we believe, will be of help to those who have trouble sleeping.

If you are worried about your sleep for any reason, getting to know more about it is a good first step towards alleviating some of that concern and breaking the vicious circle of anxiety causing loss of sleep, and worrying about loss of sleep causing more loss of sleep. In the book we shall be drawing on our experience to explain what sleep is and how it restores the mind and body; to consider the importance of dreaming and the ways in which drugs, diet and exercise affect sleep; to describe the causes and effects of lost sleep, troubled sleep and insomnia; and to offer advice on the best ways of avoiding sleeplessness.

One question we are often asked is: what makes us fall asleep? The answer tells us much about the nature of sleep, provides useful ideas for getting to sleep, and is a sensible place to begin.

# 1. WHAT MAKES US FALL ASLEEP?

First and foremost we fall asleep because we have reached that time of the twenty-four hours when we have learned to fall asleep. Many other things can, however, contribute to the ease with which we fall asleep. For example, if it is a long time since you last slept, you'll fall asleep more quickly. People who have been without sleep for two whole days and nights can drop off in a few seconds and at any time of the clock. Monotony, warmth, confinement and the satisfaction of needs, will all make us more likely to drop off.

## Our biological clock

We see patients who say they just cannot get to sleep at night and that, as a consequence, they are so tired that they feel unable to get up early in the morning. They might be surprised to find that there is a way to get up earlier. If those same people flew to India from London they would have to make a five hour change to their watches, and within a couple of weeks would largely have adjusted to the local time and conditions, and be getting up five hours earlier than they had been at home and falling asleep five hours earlier. On the first few nights in India, however, they would find it difficult to fall asleep at the local bedtime and be very sleepy when it was time to get up in the morning. By day they would be less efficient than at home and have less of a sense of well-being. The usual rhythms of their appetite for food and of their bowel movements, and, if measured, the usual daily rise and fall of body temperature across the twenty-four hours, would all be initially out of step with local time.

The social pressure weighing on them to get up earlier in India would gradually lead them to be able to fall asleep earlier and, certainly with the passage of even more weeks, their whole bodily and mental systems would adjust to the new clock time. They might still have the same trouble getting up early in India as they did in London, but they would find that they could indeed fall asleep earlier as a routine, provided they were also making a habit of getting up earlier.

## The twenty-four-hour rhythm
We all have within us a biological clock, or biorhythm, which works on an approximate twenty-four hour cycle. It is called the circadian rhythm, deriving from the Latin *circa diem*, meaning about a day. In normal life we are not much aware of it, but if we fly to the other side of the world we realize its importance and in fact it takes a couple of months for the bodily systems fully to adjust.

The very simplest forms of life, animal or vegetable, have these circadian rhythms of approximately twenty-four hours and if even small pieces of tissue are removed from the body and from their normal blood and nerve supply then, provided they receive sufficient nutrients, they will go on living and showing a circadian rhythm in the amount of oxygen they use or nutrients they take in. In the animal as a whole, the rhythmic orchestra of the tissues has a conductor, a co-ordinating centre that keeps all the body rhythms in step. It does so by means of nervous and chemical messages and is located in a small part of the brain called the suprachiasmatic nucleus. In very primitive animals this part is right up at the front end of the brain where it is most exposed to light and dark.

We shall discuss in the next chapter how living tissues are in a continual state of breakdown and at the same time a continual state of renewal. Across the day and night as a whole these two balance out, but during wakeful activity the processes of breakdown outweigh those of renewal, and during rest the processes of renewal catch up and overtake the breakdown.

For simple forms of early animal life the daylight hours meant greater warmth and consequently more movement, both for finding food and for getting into a position to be eaten, and, with the development of vision, a greater capacity for finding food. The dark phase of the twenty-four hours is, correspondingly, a cold time, a time of reduced activity, and a time for digestion of the food that has been eaten and its use for the renewal of the whole organism. It seems that over many hundreds of millions of years the capacity for changing the body's inner arrangements, according to a rhythm that approximates to the time needed for the earth to rotate on its axis – the time for changing from light and warmth to cold and darkness – has become built into the genetic constitution of every living creature. As animals evolved, some, such as the ancestors of opossums, became warm blooded and then more specialized, so that they took advantage of the relative immobility of other creatures during the dark phase and became nocturnal feeders, as is the case with most rodents and the owls that feed in turn upon them.

**Body temperature**  The circadian rhythm can very easily be demonstrated by taking someone's temperature every hour. The temperature will rise during the day and probably reach a peak during the afternoon or evening and it will decline during sleep, to reach its lowest level in the early hours of the morning.

If you stay awake all night your temperature will still fall, though it will not fall as low as it would have done had you slept. Likewise, if you continue to lie in bed all day your temperature will inevitably rise, though not to such heights as it would have done had you been physically active.

Our capacities for intellectual and bodily skill rise and fall with our temperature, as does the urge to be on the move. If you have to make arithmetical calculations, or watch a factory production-line

This graph shows both the rhythmic daily rise and fall of body temperature, and the link between body temperature and our physical and mental abilities.

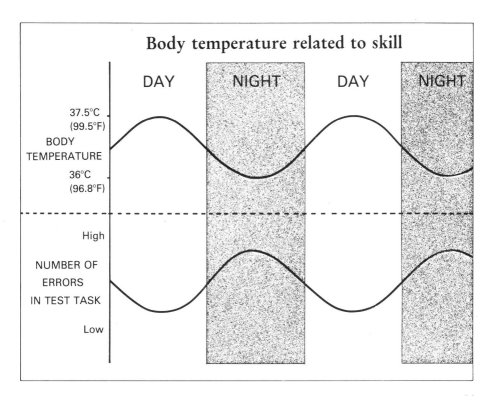

for faulty products, you will perform your job better by day when your temperature is higher and, even though awake, you will do less well at night if your temperature has fallen. Temperature and mental and physical performance are tied very closely together, as the diagram on the previous page illustrates.

**Sleepiness**   Among the other functions tied to the circadian rhythm is the feeling of sleepiness and the readiness to fall asleep. Even while being kept without sleep for several days and nights, people are more alert and lively during the time of the twenty-four hours when they are accustomed to being awake, and it is during the time when they customarily sleep that there is the greatest difficulty in staying awake.

## Keep the clock regular
People who do not stick to a regular time for going to bed and for getting up, do not have such a sharply defined rise and fall in body temperature, or rise and fall of their tendency to be sleepy. In one American study by Dr John Taub in Charlottesville, Virginia, a group of young adults, who customarily led a life in which there was variation of three or four hours from night to night in the time when they chose to go to bed, was compared with another group who were very regular in the time at which they went to bed. At the same time of day the regular people had faster reaction times, and felt themselves to be happier than those who were irregular in their sleeping habits.

Not only did the regular people feel themselves to be happier, they also had a higher opinion of the quality of their sleep and felt that they had more energy by day. It may be that some of us have a constitution that makes us into people who just don't keep regular hours and that the same basic constitution is one that makes us feel less happy and less energetic and to have a sense of poor sleep. However, it seems a reasonable guess that the irregular hours of sleep were partly a cause of feeling both less well and less pleased with life. Certainly, if irregular hours are forced on people, through shift-work, for example, many will feel that as a consequence of the irregularity of hours they are less happy, and have less energy and a poorer quality of sleep.

The same research workers in the United States did other studies using volunteers whose sleep patterns were altered. Either they were deliberately allowed to sleep three hours longer in the morning, or to go to bed three hours later and then sleep three hours later, or were put to bed three hours earlier and woken up three hours earlier.

All such deliberate interference with the normal hours of going to sleep and of waking up caused the volunteers to become slightly less efficient by day and to have less of a sense of well-being. They were at their best when they followed their normal, regular pattern of going to sleep and waking up.

That's why if you have been sleeping badly and are feeling tired and low throughout the day you should strengthen your biological clock, so that it will help you to drop off quickly to sleep at night and enable you to be really efficient by day. Sharpen it up by always going to bed at about the same time each night and always getting up at the same time in the morning.

**Why you should get up early**    The time you get up in the morning governs the time you will be feeling tired at night. So if you want to fall asleep more readily at night, then get up earlier in the morning! And do so regularly. You will get sleep of better quality and feel happier and more energetic by day if you keep it all regular.

Sixteen-year-old schoolboy Andrew Miles was sent to us for help because he couldn't fall asleep until 2 am. He was at a boarding school where lessons did not begin until about 10 am, so he never got up until 9.30 am. When he came to us we got him up regularly at 7 am each day and within a couple of weeks he was regularly fast asleep by 11 pm. If it had been the routine at his school to make the boys get up earlier, then he would have fallen asleep at a more reasonable hour each evening. Nobody would have thought him in any way peculiar and he would never have been sent to see us. It was just a matter of adjusting his circadian rhythm to a more acceptable cycle.

**Different rhythms of waking and sleeping for different people**
The term circadian rhythm means, as we have said, a rhythm of approximately twenty-four hours, but everybody is different and the innate rhythm is not precisely twenty-four hours for everybody. In most people it lasts slightly longer and in only a few as little as twenty-four hours.

You may have read accounts of people who go into underground caves and stay there for many weeks at a time for the purposes of scientific experiments. They leave their watches behind at the surface and, in total darkness, and devoid of external cues, they begin to free run, as it is called. Under these circumstances many of them will start to live a 25–hour life cycle, or even a 48–50-hour cycle and only a few will adopt a rhythm around 24 hours.

In normal life our rhythms are constantly being reset to the twenty-four hours by external factors (termed *zeitgeibers* by specialists); especially by social activity, by the morning alarm clock and getting up, by the times of meals and the alternation of light and dark. In many lower animals, such as rats, light and dark are the key factors, but in human beings social activity seems much more important.

Nevertheless, there is a greater tendency for blind people to free run on, say, a twenty-five-hour inner clock during their ordinary lives; and there are people who do not conform to society's conventions – who do not have regular work and do not care if it is night or day – who in their lives seem liable to free run. People who free run on a twenty-five-hour rhythm will get up an hour later each day and likewise will, day by day, fall asleep one hour later and wake up an hour later and another hour later, until they are not sleeping at all during conventional hours, but sleep during the day. Days later

Your body's rhythms for going to sleep and waking up are continually being adjusted by external factors such as the morning alarm clock.

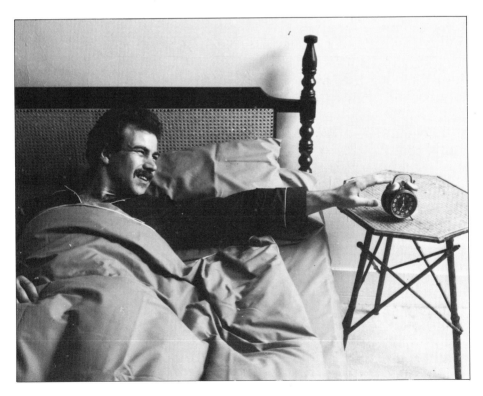

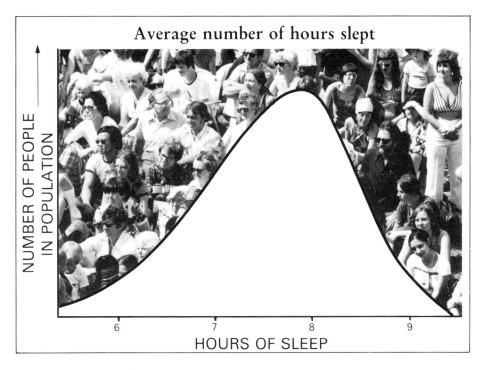

## Average number of hours slept

*NUMBER OF PEOPLE IN POPULATION*

6      7      8      9

**HOURS OF SLEEP**

A few people need just six hours sleep each night, a few sleep for nine hours, but most have around seven to eight hours sleep.

they will again start to become sleepy in the evenings and wakeful in the mornings. This cycle will continue so that they get into step with the rest of their countrymen and out of step, into step and out of step again about every twenty-five days.

It is because we are all sensitive to a different degree to the external factors – the *zeitgeibers* – that influence our waking and sleeping habits, and because we all differ in our tendency to free run that we also differ in how easy we feel it is to fall asleep at a precise and regular evening hour, and how easy it is to feel wakeful and alert at a precise and regular morning hour. In fact, in any human activity, or anything else in the world of biology, it is important to remember the wide individual variations. Some people have big feet and some have small feet: but most people's are in the middle. Some people sleep for a long time and others for a short time: most people are in the middle. Some find it easy always to fall asleep at night and others find it difficult: again, most people are in the middle. As a general rule, though, if you stick firmly to regular hours you can help your own inner clock to keep regular habits.

# What else makes us sleep?

## Lack of sleep

Everyone knows that if you have little sleep one night, then the following day you are more likely to drop off in the afternoon or early in the evening. In the early 1970s, two American psychologists in Gainesville, Florida, measured the time taken between settling to sleep and actually dropping off and showed that it did indeed get shorter and shorter according to the number of hours since the volunteers last slept. It means that if you are very short of sleep you would be unwise to take on tasks such as prolonged driving on motorways and freeways where you might fall asleep without warning and have an accident.

## Monotony and other causes

Motorway and freeway driving is a well-known cause of sleepiness and it's the monotony that's the principal reason.

A few years ago a British motoring magazine published a discussion about falling asleep when driving, together with the results of a survey by the police in the county of Cumbria, in the north of England. The M6 motorway runs from London, northwards through the industrial regions of the Midlands and Lancashire, and then continues through the beautiful stretches of the Cumbrian countryside. The route through the industrial areas is always busy, with cars and trucks moving in and out, so that there is always plenty to keep drivers awake. In Cumbria there are long empty stretches where a driver might scarcely see another vehicle, and monotony and the tiredness caused by a long journey can often become overwhelming. The Cumbrian police found that around 25 per cent of accidents seemed to have been caused by motorists falling asleep at the wheel and simply driving off the road at a shallow angle, without leaving any tyre marks on the road surface.

You can understand the effects of monotony more easily if you consider how anything new or exciting alerts you and prevents you falling asleep. Novelty will keep you awake, and by contrast the uniformity that monotony imposes will predispose you to sleep. We have demonstrated this in our laboratory by comparing the liability to fall asleep of volunteers who simply lie in bed doing nothing in particular, with the liability of others who are deliberately subjected to monotonous hooting noises. We found that the monotonous noises made people fall asleep more quickly, and this explains the use of rhythmic sounds such as the noise of waves on the sea shore or noises like heartbeats to help people who feel they have difficulty in getting to sleep at night.

Knowing that monotony brings sleep more quickly is useful to parents of wakeful young babies. If, once you have attended to all your healthy baby's basic needs – feeding, a clean nappy or diaper, and warmth – and you still have trouble getting him or her off to sleep, rocking the baby either in a pram or your arms will often do the trick. And many parents find playing monotonous music or singing repetitive lullabies have the same effect.

Obviously, when you are walking about, you are less likely to fall asleep than when sitting still. Immobility and confinement in a small car, for example, or in the cabin of a truck on a highway, again contribute to the tendency to fall asleep. The same is true of warmth. If you feel cold, your muscles become more tense and you may even shiver, all of which is a mechanism for maintaining your best temperature but it tends at the same time to keep you awake. When you

Rocking a baby is a good example of how rhythmic monotony tends to bring on sleep.

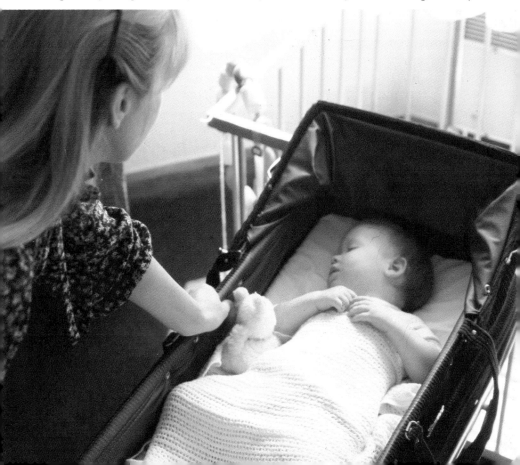

feel warm your muscles relax and sleep comes more easily; a good reason to make sure your bedroom is warm and that you have sufficient bedclothes during the cold winter months. Satisfaction of important needs is also followed by relaxation and a greater tendency to sleepiness. Many of us will fall asleep more readily after a good meal or sexual intercourse.

# What happens as we fall asleep?

### The 100-minute rhythm
There is no sudden or sharp division between being awake and being asleep. When awake, we can become more and more relaxed and engage in what we call day-dreaming, and at these moments our brains are functioning in a state that approaches that of obvious drowsiness. The day-dreaminess can actually come and go rhythmically, every 100 minutes. In the next chapter we shall describe how during the night our sleep alternates between two different states about once every 100 minutes. It is an example of yet another biological rhythm, and is present in us while we are awake as well. This rhythm is known as an ultradian rhythm.

Generally we are so involved in our social activities that we are quite unaware of the rhythm, but on our own, in a dull and boring situation where we have nothing to do, research has shown that we become more restless and less restless, more restless and less restless about every 100 minutes. We are also more inclined to nibble any available food about once every 100 minutes, and to drowse slightly and engage in day-dreaming, on and off, according to the same rhythm. We now know that alertness and drowsiness can come and go not only according to the twenty-four-hour circadian rhythm but according to this 100-minute ultradian rhythm too.

### Dropping off
One of the grandfathers of American psychiatry, Dr Weir Mitchell, famous for treating the nervous disorders of soldiers in the Civil War by a regime of total rest, was very interested in disorders of sleep and in the events of drowsiness. He described how, while we fall asleep, the control of our ideas escapes us as we drowse, and we begin to live in a world apart. The drowsier we are, the more that world gets separated from the real world around us. Especially if we are in the dark, we begin to have little dreams in which we see events and people that are not really there. We engage in fantasy conver-

sations with our dream companions, we seem to hear our own voice speaking to them and them replying to us. Abruptly, we may make a return to full reality and to alert wakefulness, but if it is in the late evening and our normal time for going to sleep, then our grip upon reality becomes more tenuous, our little dream experiences become more vivid, we slip further into sleep and when we do suddenly rouse for a moment, wakened by what Mitchell described as a sensory shock, it may be with a sudden jerk.

The voices and visions and other sensations of falling asleep are termed hypnagogic (or leading-to-sleep) hallucinations. They are entirely normal and nothing to be concerned about; usually we forget them completely. If you think you don't have them, and are interested to find out, then get someone to wake you up just as you are dropping off to sleep, or train yourself to do so, and immediately write down what you have just been experiencing. You will find that you have often been hearing your own voice saying some extraordinary phrase, perhaps with strange words that do not really exist.

The father of modern European psychiatry, Dr Emil Kraepelin of Germany, was very interested in these irrational moments when we briefly lose touch. He was a great collector of the strange phrases of drowsiness. Among the hundreds of examples that Kraepelin published while working in Munich can be found phrases as strange as: 'Lord string-player and muscle sardines'. Some of the oddest from our own collection are: 'Or squawns of medication allow me to ungather', and: 'Only God and Henry Ford have no umbilical cord.'

Although it's unusual to remember these phrases, if you ask people at a social gathering if they have ever suddenly woken up thinking that their name had been called aloud, there will be many who will acknowledge this experience; and a few who will describe how they had woken up and seen an angel, or someone else in the room, and then a few moments later had realized that they were now fully awake and that the apparition was no longer there. Generally the visions and voices of drowsiness are not frightening, but if we are in a general state of anxiety or fever, then the visions and voices can form themselves into frightening phantoms. They are, though, nothing more than phantoms from our own drowsy minds. We will be looking in more detail at the whole question of dreaming in Chapter 4. But first, now you know more about falling asleep, it is time to find out how your mind and body are refreshed and restored during sleep.

# 2. SLEEP, THE GREAT RESTORER

In our busy world of waking life we literally burn up our tissues faster than we renew them. Living tissues are being worn out and renewed all the time, and across an average twenty-four hours we keep the two processes in balance. The wearing out and the renewal continue both by day and by night; but the wearing out is more predominant by day, and the renewal by night.

It is not only so many hours of sleep we need, we need sleep of good, refreshing quality. Most people feel refreshed by their sleep. But others are less fortunate and feel that somehow they are not fully restored by their night's sleep; they feel less vigorous by day; and feel that their cares have remained with them throughout the night.

We can record the electrical brain waves of volunteers with this problem, and in fact most of them differ little in their hours spent asleep and the number of times they wake up from most other people of their own age. In the last few years, however, we have begun to make measurements of just how restorative sleep may be, and it looks as though many of the people who feel that they sleep poorly, although they may sleep as long as other people, really do have less of the kind of sleep that restores; at least as far as we can judge from their hormones. Some poor sleepers, for example, have unusually high night-time levels of the hormones that hinder the renewal of brain and body tissues.

## How hormones affect the quality of sleep

The scientist always wants to make objective measurements. Tiny pieces of skin can be cut off and the rate at which the skin cells are multiplying and renewing themselves at any one time can then be measured. Sure enough, human skin cells renew themselves faster during the time of sleep. The same seems to be true of human blood cells. And we know from studies with animals that every tissue of the body from the brain to the sole of the foot renews its structure faster during sleep.

What we can do in human beings, is to try and understand the body's controls of the restorative function of sleep. Very important are the hormones, or chemical messengers, of which very small amounts circulate in our blood. Some of these hormones come from the pituitary gland at the base of the brain and their release into the blood is controlled by the workings of the brain. Other important hormones are released from the adrenal glands, which are situated just above the kidneys.

## The hormones of wakefulness

**Adrenaline (epinephrine)** This is one very important hormone released from the adrenal glands in large amounts while we are awake, but hardly at all while we sleep. Small quantities of adrenaline are present in the blood all the time that we are awake, but in moments when there are extra demands upon us, and most of all when we are under stress or frightened, the adrenaline rises to high levels. It enables our muscles to exert greater power, using up enormous quantities of their energy reserves in a very short space of time.

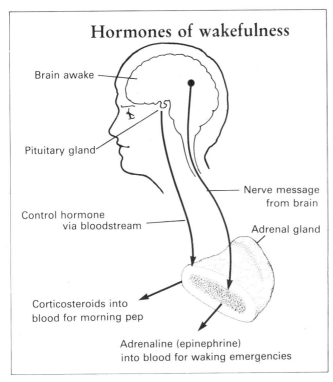

### Hormones of wakefulness

Brain awake

Pituitary gland

Nerve message from brain

Control hormone via bloodstream

Adrenal gland

Corticosteroids into blood for morning pep

Adrenaline (epinephrine) into blood for waking emergencies

The hormones of wakefulness – adrenaline (epinephrine) and corticosteroids – give us pep to cope with emergencies while we are awake, but hinder the renewal of the body's tissues. They are released into the bloodstream from the adrenal glands, near the kidneys. The adrenaline is triggered by nerve messages from the brain; the corticosteroids, by a control hormone from the pituitary gland.

Dealing with emergencies takes priority over everything else. In emergencies the body is heedless of wearing out the tissues at a faster rate, and holds in abeyance the processes of restoration, including the digestion of food and the eventual use of food materials for rebuilding the body. It is not just the muscles that are working with greater force during emergencies, giving priority to needs other than the manufacture of the proteins – the building blocks that make up the structure of the tissue – the same things are happening in the brain too, as far as we can judge.

Adrenaline positively inhibits the formation of new protein in tissues and this fact by itself makes wakefulness a time of reduced manufacture of what is needed to keep the tissues renewed compared with the time of sleep. Adrenaline has a close relative, a hormone called noradrenaline (norepinephrine), and the amount of this in the brain is greater by day and helps us to be more effective in dealing with problems, but it too reduces protein renewal.

**Corticosteroids** The adrenal glands release other hormones into the bloodstream that are called corticosteroids. These corticosteroids seem to complement the adrenaline by providing a sort of steadying back-up influence. Although adrenaline is being released all the time and especially while we are awake, it comes in sudden high-intensity spurts according to the moment-to-moment challenges that we face. In contrast, the corticosteroids provide a general background to improve our waking capacities. They are almost absent during the early night, but towards the later part of the night's sleep they begin to be found in larger quantities in the blood, until they reach very high levels soon after our usual time for waking up. They seem like a morning tonic, a sort of pick-me-up that is not needed so much during the afternoon and evening. The corticosteroids too, like adrenaline, positively inhibit the manufacture of the new protein that is necessary for tissue renewal.

We can see then that the main hormones of wakefulness, while they are very important in enabling us to meet the demands of the day, also ensure that achievement while we are awake has priority over providing balm to our minds or renewal to our bodies.

### The restoring hormones of sleep
When we go to sleep, the renewal of the body's tissue, provided by the manufacture of fresh protein, can proceed faster; and not merely because of the relative absence of the waking hormones, adrenaline and corticosteroids, but because manufacture is positively encour-

aged by the presence of new hormones released into the bloodstream while we are asleep. There are several of these body-building, or anabolic, hormones. Testosterone, a male hormone, is perhaps best known as a body-building hormone that has been used illegally in attempts to interfere with Nature and enable international athletes to perform with greater prowess; and testosterone is among the hormones that rise in concentration in the blood during sleep. Among the others is a hormone that is known as growth hormone. Growth hormone really does what it says, it makes tissue grow faster.

**Growth hormone** The manufacture of new protein material for growing taller is the same process as the manufacture of new protein material for the replacement of what has been worn out by activity during the day. Growth hormone is released by the pituitary gland when it is told by the brain that sleep is present. The mechanism is a very old one in evolutionary terms, for it has been discovered to exist in fishes. As a consequence, although there is quite a lot of growth hormone in the blood while we are awake, the amounts are much higher during sleep. If you were to go without sleep for a

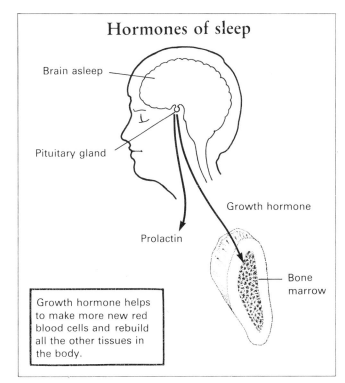

## Hormones of sleep

Brain asleep

Pituitary gland

Growth hormone

Prolactin

Bone marrow

Growth hormone helps to make more new red blood cells and rebuild all the other tissues in the body.

The hormones released by the pituitary gland into the bloodstream when we sleep encourage the renewal of body tissue that has been worn out during the day.

couple of days, when at last you fell asleep, the growth hormone would really rush out into your bloodstream to help the renewal of the tissues.

Helped by the low levels of the daytime hormones – adrenaline (epinephrine) and the corticosteroids – while we sleep, the body-building hormones, like growth hormone, really can do their best for us at the time of sleep. It has actually been found that in children who have a deficiency of growth hormone, the growth processes can better be helped by giving an injection of growth hormone just before they sleep than by giving the same amount of growth hormone as an injection at breakfast time.

Although we have said a lot about the hormones, they are only part of the chemical system controlling the body's renewal. Very simple forms of life that do not have hormones circulating in the bloodstream, but which take in food during the daylight hours and rest during darkness, also have a predominance of protein manufacture and tissue renewal during their times of rest, and this is because when the living cells of either simple creatures or complex ones like ourselves are using up a lot of energy on moving around, the cells of the body are not geared for making protein or for restoration, and it is only when the energy levels within the cells can rise through rest, that renewal can again take place.

# Unrefreshing sleep: the hormones working at cross-purposes

We have already explained about our biological clocks and have emphasized that the keeping of regular hours for going to bed and getting up helps sleep to feel good and people to feel happier and more energetic by day. This is because regular hours help to keep the hormones of sleep and wakefulness operating in harmony – that is, each working with each other and at the time of the twenty-four hours when each can best perform its particular function.

It is common to have a night's sleep after which you feel tired and unrefreshed; the cause may be partly traced to the keeping of irregular hours. This can disturb the biological clock and make the two sets of hormones work counterproductively, at cross-purposes. The occasional late night does not cause any long-term problem with the balanced working of these hormones, but many people nowadays have jobs that require them to lead an unnatural life for getting up

24

and going to work. A close look at their sleeping patterns tells us about the way hormones can make sleep unrefreshing.

## Shift-work

Aircrew have to fly around the world and keep changing their pattern of life, their times for eating and for going to bed and getting up, according to local clock times. Nurses and policemen have always had to sacrifice conventional hours of eating and sleeping and for being with their families; and nowadays, when it may be wasteful not to keep expensive industrial machinery in use steadily around the clock, a higher proportion of the population is called upon to undertake shift-work.

In theory, if you worked a regular night-shift you could change your whole pattern of life and readjust your biological clock so that you got your highest temperature at night and your lowest by day, and then you would be just as bright and efficient at night as you are by day while you lead a regular life of daytime work. In practice

Working night-shifts disturbs the balanced working of the hormones of sleep and wake-fulness. As a result, many shift-workers feel less refreshed by their sleep.

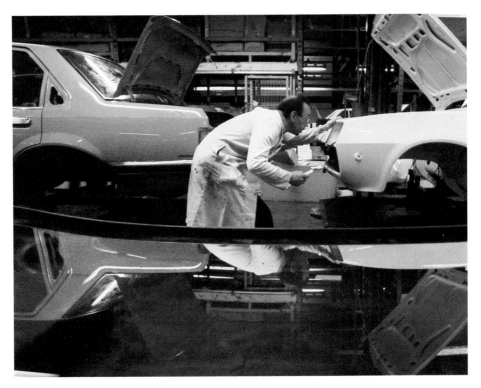

this does not happen, because people have days off, and on those days they like to mingle with their families and friends, go to social events, and do all the other things that their family and friends are doing during the day. As a consequence shift-workers never really make a full adjustment to any kind of regular twenty-four-hour pattern. Different individuals react differently to shift-work, but for some it is certainly a cause of feeling below par both physically and emotionally.

If you look at the diagram you can understand better how shift-work makes it more difficult for the body to give us good, restful and restorative sleep. In the first place it may be difficult to get to sleep at the unnatural time – perhaps with strong daylight and noisy children – and what sleep comes is more likely to be disturbed by noisier conditions. A look at the hormone arrangements within the body shows that the daytime hormones, the corticosteroids and the adrenaline that favour breakdown of tissues and not their renewal, rise and fall every twenty-four hours according to a circadian rhythm. If you suddenly go on to night-shift, then the adrenaline and the

The night-shift changes the rhythm of the sleep hormones. Consequently, their restorative effect during sleep the next day is reduced by the high levels of adrenaline and corticosteroids, whose rise is governed by a twenty-four-hour cycle, not by being awake or asleep.

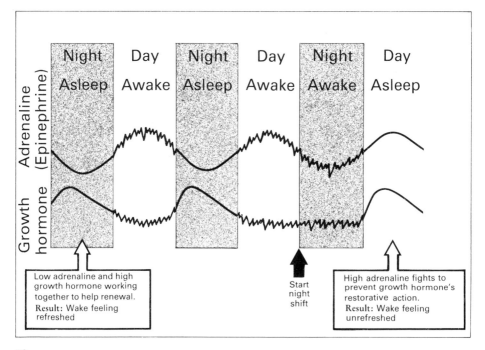

corticosteroids will not rise quite as high during the day while you are doing your best to sleep, but rise they inevitably will. Weeks of a regular routine would be needed to switch them round completely to being low by day when the night-shift worker would be hoping to sleep; and in practice, as we have said, this does not happen because of the demands of family and social life.

The body-building hormones of sleep, however, are not governed by a circadian rhythm but by sleep itself. Just by going to bed and lying down does not mean that more growth hormone will be released into your bloodstream. You have got to sleep, and sleep deeply. When therefore you go on to night-shift working and go to bed at 9 am, provided you fall into a deep sleep, the growth hormone will certainly be released into your blood, but now its good effects will be counteracted all the time you are asleep by the high levels of adrenaline and corticosteroids in the blood which would not have been there had your deep sleep and your growth hormone come to you in the middle of the night. Normally we have a very sensible relationship such that the hormones that favour lively achievement and inhibit the renewal of body tissues are kept out of the way while we sleep. Evolution did not include shift-work rotas.

Earlier we said that individuals differ, and some people do find it more difficult to adjust to shift-work. Middle-aged and older people fall less easily into sound sleep at any time than young people, and they are also less adaptable in facing sudden clock changes if they fly around the world, and again they find it less easy to get satisfactory sleep if they go on to shift-work. Broad generalizations like these do not apply to everyone; you may be able to point to someone among your friends who is middle-aged and finds no problem at all in being a shift-worker, but he may be just the lucky exception.

All life is a compromise and we have to accept the disadvantages as well as the benefits of our modern society. We are not advocating that people stop doing shift-work, but we do urge that there should be a better understanding of the difficulties that some people face when they are asked to cope with shift-work. They may become not only less vigorous, but also less efficient, less happy and less emotionally stable. They should not be condemned out of hand; it may just be that they have stricter biological clocks and hormone systems.

Once you have entered the routine of shift-work there is little you can do to counter the unwanted effects of your hormones working at cross-purposes; there are no medicines that will help. One thing that will make their effects worse, and which should be avoided, is heavy consumption of alcohol.

# 3.  MEASURING SLEEP

## Methods of measurement

If we are going to try and understand sleep better, then we have got
to be able to make measurements. There are four common methods
researchers use for measuring the sleep of volunteers. First, each can
say in the morning how many hours they believe they must have
slept, or how good a quality of sleep they feel they had. Then, if
they are in hospital, a nurse can come along every half an hour and
make a note of whether she thinks they are awake or asleep (but,
you may ask, will she wake them up by giving such a lot of attention?). We move less when we are asleep, and so another method of
measurement is provided by the number of movements made or how
much energy is put into them. The fourth, and most expensive but
most refined approach is to make a record throughout the night of
the electrical brain waves, and to see for what proportion of time the
waves show the signs of sleep.

### Personal estimation
The personal and subjective estimation of how many hours and
minutes you have slept is easily enough done, but many research
investigations have shown that volunteers are not very accurate in
estimating the duration of their own sleep, to judge by the more
exact measurements of how much sleep they got according to the
electrical brain-wave records. In many of the research studies at our
laboratory we have asked people to make an estimate or rating of
the quality of the sleep they had had during the preceding night and
to do this they filled in each morning what is known as a visual
analogue scale (see opposite).

The method is a cheap one, and is acceptable to most people, who
are willing to fill in these rating scales every morning for many
months. In the end, the number of millimetres between the left-hand
end of the scale and the mark that they have made in the morning
can be measured.

In one test we gave volunteers pills regularly at bedtime, which,

# The visual analogue scale

**QUALITY OF SLEEP**
Please make a mark on the line to indicate how well or how badly you feel you slept last night. A mark in the centre would mean an average, normal night, a mark to the left a poor night, a mark to the right a better night.

Worst
possible _____ Best ever

The visual analogue scale is used by researchers to gauge the quality of volunteers' sleep. The volunteer makes a mark on the horizontal line according to how well he feels he has slept.

without their knowledge, were suddenly switched from inactive pills to identical-looking ones containing one of the more usual sleeping drugs. The visual analogue scale ratings at once told us that the volunteers thought they were sleeping better. When, after some months of nightly intake of the pills containing the drug, the pills were again changed, and this time back to the original identical-looking but inactive pills, then they felt that they were at first sleeping very badly indeed, and the measurements in millimetres on the visual analogue scales at once betrayed this.

## An observer's estimation
A similar use can be made of nurses' judgements. Occasionally people claim that they have hardly slept a wink for many years. The great majority feel that they are being deprived of something that they wish they could enjoy more of, and are concerned about what they feel is a lack of sleep. We and many other sleep researchers have studied the sleep of such people; and if you share this problem you

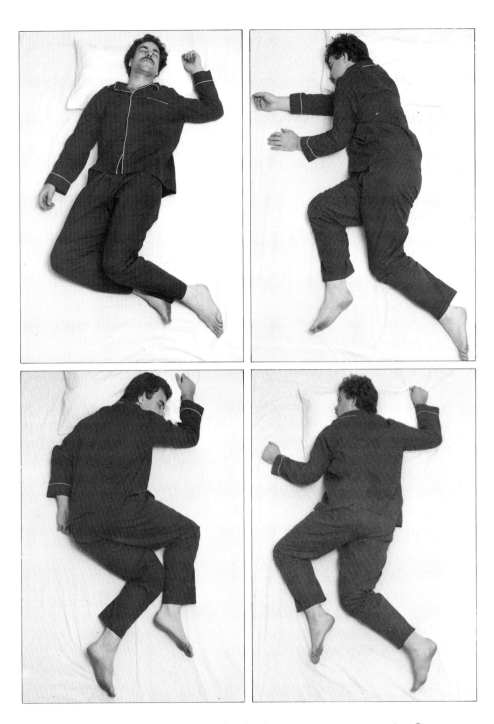

Generally, the more restful your sleep is, the less movements you make. On average, you change position about forty to fifty times a night.

may be surprised and reassured by what we found. Simple observation alone, such as a nurse can make, invariably confirmed that such people actually are asleep nearly the whole night, perhaps snoring, with every appearance of continued slumber and quite unaware of the presence of the observer.

## Recording body movement

It is possible to use a small device rather like one of those wristwatches that are self-winding, and in which a weight is moved in position whenever the wearer's arm moves, to make a record of the body's activity. The movement of the weight alters a counter and so gives, over a period of time, a rough indication of the number and vigour of movements.

Such measurements of body movements are not very reliable for telling us the point at which somebody fell asleep, because obviously you can be awake and lie absolutely still for quite long periods. Some people move frequently while they are asleep and others rarely, so that the method is not very precise for telling us whether any one person has been asleep during any particular period of the night. Taking the measurements for a group of people all together, however, the method gives a good general indication of the most restful times.

## The electroencephalograph (EEG)

Electrical brain waves can be measured because the brain operates by chemical and electrical means. It is made up of tiny units, called cells, surrounded by fluid; and the chemical constitution within the cells differs from the chemicals in the surrounding fluid. Just as a battery that we put into a torch will produce small electric currents because of the chemicals it contains, so the cells in the brain generate tiny electrical currents.

Over the head as a whole the electricity from the millions of cells in the brain is joined together. If, therefore, small silver discs are fixed to the scalp, and wires are then led from those discs into a sensitive machine for measuring electricity, the machine can show us the variations in how the cells are working in the form of electrical brain waves, or the electroencephalogram.

The machine that we use, called an electroencephalograph (EEG), is really a very delicate and expensive voltmeter. Instead of having a needle on a scale, ink flows from the tips of fine pens on to paper, so that when the needle-pens make movements the electrical brain waves are written out as ink traces upon moving paper (see page 34). If we arrange for there to be an endless supply of paper, made up of individual pages separated by perforations, and if each of those pages takes twenty seconds to run through, then we can say how many pages (thus minutes) of paper flowed during the time between lights-out and first falling asleep. Again, by studying the shapes and patterns of the waves we can say how much time was spent in wakefulness, and in which parts of the night it occurred; and we can also say how many minutes were spent in which stages of sleep.

# The stages and types of sleep

The appearance of the electrical brain waves varies according to whether we are brightly alert, quietly relaxed, peacefully drowsy, or soundly asleep. When we are awake and relaxed, especially if our eyes are closed, we often have brain rhythms at about 10 waves per second; these waves we call the alpha rhythm. The alpha rhythm disappears if we face a sudden and new challenge in life, particularly if the eyes are open at the same time. The rhythm also disappears when we become drowsy and it then becomes replaced by rather slower waves. We call the brain waves of drowsiness, stage 1 sleep. If we are really going to sleep, then we go into stage 2 sleep, in which the electrical brain waves are quite a lot slower and in which some distinctively shaped waves called spindles make their appearance (see diagram on page 34). In young people, and especially in the early part of the night, stage 2 will progress to brain waves with more and more large slow waves and we call this pattern stage 3, or, with even more slow waves, stage 4. All these four stages are termed 'orthodox' sleep. Interspersed with orthodox sleep is another phase of sleep we have not yet mentioned, namely 'paradoxical', or rapid eye movement (REM), sleep.

### Orthodox and paradoxical sleep

Paradoxical and orthodox, or non-rapid eye movement (NREM), sleep alternate throughout the night, governed by the 100-minute ultradian rhythm. Normally, about 20 per cent of sleep is paradoxical and 80 per cent orthodox. The recorded brain waves of paradoxical sleep are smaller and faster than those of the deeper stages of orthodox sleep and in fact resemble those of drowsiness. The tell-tale movements of the eyes can also be detected using the EEG because the machine can be set up to record movements of the eyeballs as well as electrical brain rhythms.

However, the existence of this kind of sleep was first observed

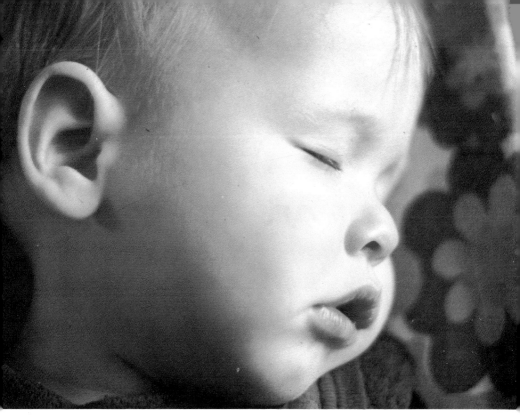

Babies spend a great deal of their sleeping life in paradoxical or rapid eye movement (REM) sleep.

without the aid of an EEG simply by watching babies and seeing that for some periods during their sleep their eyes were jerking hither and thither for minutes on end. When paradoxical sleep was first being described, it was not then realized that it was a different kind of sleep, and it was thought of as light sleep with dreaming. Later it was found to be accompanied by the greatest muscle relaxation, as if it were the deepest sleep, at the same time as being the lightest sleep – hence the name 'paradoxical'. Many journalists fostered the idea that it was 'dreaming sleep' and the additional notion that we had to have it in order to remain sane. The latter suggestion we know to be untrue, and we now realize that we can dream during all other stages of sleep, though we recognize that the richest dreams are experienced during paradoxical sleep.

Really it is wrong to think of either paradoxical or orthodox sleep as being the deeper or lighter. In stage 4 of orthodox sleep we are most difficult to awaken; but in paradoxical sleep our muscles are at their most relaxed, so that you could say that either of these types

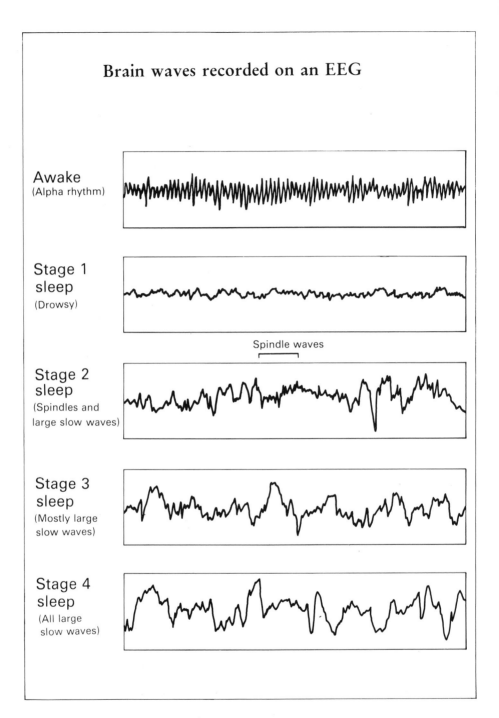

Brain waves recorded on an EEG

**Awake**
(Alpha rhythm)

**Stage 1 sleep**
(Drowsy)

Spindle waves

**Stage 2 sleep**
(Spindles and large slow waves)

**Stage 3 sleep**
(Mostly large slow waves)

**Stage 4 sleep**
(All large slow waves)

These lines are sections from an EEG print-out. Each of the bottom four brain-wave patterns is distinctive of a particular stage of sleep.

# Normal proportions of orthodox and paradoxical sleep

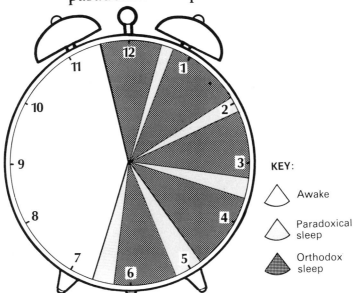

**KEY:**

△ Awake

△ Paradoxical sleep

▲ Orthodox sleep

Orthodox or NREM sleep alternates with paradoxical or REM sleep throughout the night. Taking sleeping drugs or alcohol will alter these proportions.

of sleep is the deeper, depending upon what you think is the more important. The fact is that they are just different. In paradoxical sleep we have twitching movements, not only of the eyeballs, but of many parts of the body. Cats or dogs will twitch their tails, their whiskers, and the tips of their paws so that we will say, 'That dog's dreaming.' We too twitch our faces; and our breathing, heartbeat and blood pressure become irregular; a remarkable paralysis affects most of our body except for those momentary twitches; and the blood rushes through the brain at a faster rate than during orthodox sleep. During paradoxical sleep too, whether sexual dreams are being experienced or not, in men the penis becomes erect, and in women the blood flows more rapidly around the vagina, while the nipples become erect. The paralysis of the muscles in paradoxical sleep forms the basis for the occasional experience that any of us can have of waking from a dream and momentarily feeling unable to move.

It seems likely that paradoxical sleep is actually the oldest kind of sleep in evolutionary terms, for it is a time when the brain no longer keeps the body's temperature constant by making muscles shiver and it seems to be the sleep of our ancient cold-blooded ancestors. Orthodox slow-wave sleep is in some ways certainly more restorative (it is the stage when growth hormone is released into the bloodstream); and is probably a necessity for warm-blooded creatures like ourselves, who expend vastly more energy while we are awake than do cold-blooded reptiles. In the course of evolution, some warm-blooded animals have evolved a particular kind of orthodox sleep, with very slow electrical brain waves, in which their body temperature falls even more than it does during our sleep, down to very low levels; and they then expend hardly any energy in keeping themselves alive. This is hibernation.

### Does it matter if you don't get enough paradoxical sleep?

We are not able to say that for human beings the one kind of sleep or the other is in any way better, and there is no evidence that lack of paradoxical sleep will leave us unrefreshed. We just need sleep, and we need both kinds of sleep. The proportions or amounts that we get of each are beyond our own control. Drugs will change the proportions, and most drugs, such as sleeping drugs, reduce the time spent in paradoxical sleep. Although this reduction is a departure from normal, it does not mean that we are going to come to harm as a result. Do not believe anybody who tells you that you ought to have more paradoxical sleep with its rapid eye movements. Left to itself, the brain can look after its own needs, so long as we do not insult it too much by keeping grossly irregular hours, or by excessive indulgence in alcohol or other drugs.

Many disturbing misconceptions have arisen over the years about the need for the different types of sleep and especially about their connection with dreaming. Dreams and nightmares are the subject of the next chapter, in which we will be attempting to dispel some of the myths.

# 4. DREAMS AND NIGHTMARES

In the course of our work we are often asked about dreaming: whether dreams have any ulterior significance, whether we all dream every night, whether we will come to any harm if we don't dream, whether having nightmares means that we are psychologically disturbed, and so on. As we will be showing in this chapter, scientific research has provided answers to many of these and other common related questions.

The central area of Fuseli's *The Shepherd's Dream* (1793) shows the dreamer in the middle of his supernatural fantasy world. Compare with his picture on page 44.

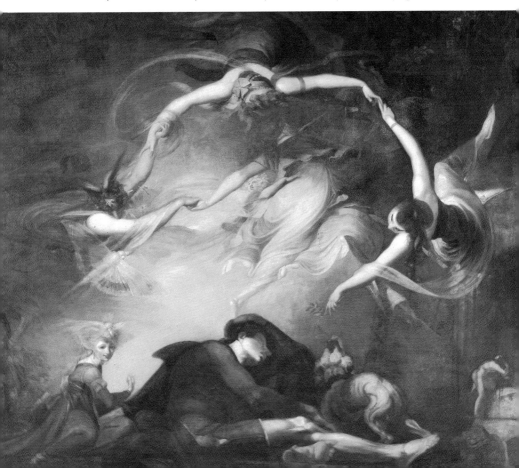

# What happens when we dream?

Your dreams may be fascinating, frightening or puzzling, though most often just plain dull; but whatever they are, they soon melt into thin air. A dream is a fantasy, a living in an unreal world, seeing things that are not really there, experiencing emotions, mingling with people, right there in the middle of a living fantasy world, and not being a passive observer watching some flickering screen. Interestingly, people who have been blind from birth see nothing in their dreams, but still dream as vividly as you or I while living in their fantasy world.

This fantasy world, which we all share, has been the subject of speculation and superstition from earliest times. As far back as records go, and all around the world, there have been beliefs linking dreams with the supernatural; dreams have been considered prophetic; and right down the centuries to the present day, people have used dreams as a means of fortune-telling.

It was not until the turn of this century, however, that dreams were considered in a more scientific and analytic way. In 1901 Sigmund Freud published *The Interpretation of Dreams*, the book that he always believed to have been his greatest work. In it he described the history of ideas about dreams and set forward his own, that were very much in keeping with the beliefs of many other writers of the late nineteenth century. Freud added a particular belief in sexual symbolism and came to believe that dreams were the 'royal road to the unconscious' by which the dreamer's basic personality traits might best be understood.

His contemporary and sometime follower, Carl Gustav Jung (a man of gentler and somewhat mystical outlook), was no less impressed by the importance of dreams. He saw us as striving in our waking world to be tough and successful, and at the same time repressing the need we all feel to express our artistic and more visionary selves. It was through our dreams, Jung believed, that this other half or 'shadow' could find expression.

## When and how often do we dream?

Laboratory research into dreams really established itself during the 1950s and 1960s. Dr Nathaniel Kleitman in Chicago with his research students, Drs Aserinski and Dement, had noticed the jerking movements of the eyeballs that we now recognize to be part of the picture of paradoxical sleep. Perhaps, they thought, these are the eyes looking around at the visual events of the dreams. Kleitman and Dement tried waking people up from sleep when their eyeballs had just been jerking around and asked if they had just been dreaming. In 80 per cent of cases 'yes' was the answer; whereas when the awakenings were made from times of sleep without the jerking eyeballs, in other words from orthodox sleep, only 7 per cent said they had been dreaming.

You may be one of those who say they never dream, but laboratory research has shown that everyone does indeed dream, that some people rapidly forget, and that only if questioned almost immediately after awakening from paradoxical sleep will the dream be remembered. Some people who say that they never dream will say that they have been 'thinking' during their sleep, and when asked what they have been thinking about ('I was thinking that I was sitting on an elephant on the top of a yellow bus') it becomes obvious that a great deal depends upon what the word 'dream' means to different people.

Realizing this, Dr David Foulkes, in the United States, stopped using the word 'dream' in his questions. Waking volunteers up from sleep, he simply asked, 'Was anything passing through your mind?' Again the thoroughgoing dreams with wild fantasies were almost always described after awakenings from paradoxical sleep, but many awakenings from paradoxical sleep also yielded dull and prosaic accounts related to waking life that differed little from the accounts given after awakenings from orthodox sleep.

The early days of laboratory dream research revealed how quickly the memory of a dream is lost if it is not immediately recalled. When it was also discovered that the periods with rapid eye movements lasted almost two hours every night, there was a mistaken tendency to equate dreaming with periods of rapid eye movements and to assume that dreaming did not occur at other times, although it had really been known for a long time that dreams could also occur when first falling asleep, long before the first episode of paradoxical sleep of the night. The subsequent work of David Foulkes confirmed that many adventurous dreams with rich fantasy can occur during the time when we first fall asleep at night, though generally the time is not such a rich mine of experiences as the later periods of paradoxical sleep.

# Our psychological need to dream

While the ancients thought that dreams gave opportunities to mingle with supernatural beings, the psychoanalytic writers of the twentieth century have assumed that dreams have some other important function for psychological health. In *The Interpretation of Dreams* Freud wrote: 'The unconscious impulse is the real creator of the dream. . . . Just like any other instinctual impulse it can do no other but seek its own satisfaction, and our experience in dream interpretation shows us, moreover, that this is the meaning of all dreaming. In every dream an instinctual wish is displayed as fulfilled.' Later Freud wrote that dreams 'are the guardians of sleep and not its disturbers. Either the mind pays no attention at all to occasions for sensation during sleep . . . or it makes use of a dream in order to deny the stimuli.'

Freud therefore saw dreams as serving definite psychic functions. Within the unconscious mind, in his view, were imperious, earthy urges that could not be denied; and satisfaction of these impulses, too reprehensible for waking life, could be allowed during sleep in the form of dreams. It was by what he called 'dream-work' that the impulses of the unconscious mind could receive disguised satisfaction without disgrace or shame. The dream also served to disguise outside events received by the sense organs during sleep and so sheltered the sleeper from reality.

### Will lack of dreams harm you?

In the late 1950s, with these theories in mind, a New York psychoanalyst of unusually experimental bent, and with a particular interest in dreams, Dr Charles Fisher, invited the young Dr William Dement, who had earlier worked with Kleitman, to come to New York and conduct some new research into dreams. As a psychoanalyst, Dr Fisher believed there to be important psychological functions for dreaming and, with dreaming at that time mistakenly being more or less equated with periods of paradoxical sleep, Dr Dement set out to deprive people of their dreams to see what might then happen.

Normally, when people fall asleep from having been awake, they always pass first into orthodox sleep. Therefore, by waking people up each time they entered the paradoxical phase of sleep with rapid eye movements, and keeping them awake for a couple of minutes, followed by a return always into orthodox sleep initially, Dement was able selectively to deprive volunteers of paradoxical sleep and, as he believed at the time, to deprive them of dreams. He did this on five successive nights and, as the nights followed one another, the awakenings had to become more and more frequent, as if the volunteers were attempting more and more urgently to get back to their dreams. When finally allowed to sleep undisturbed, the volunteers spent more time than normal in the paradoxical phase of sleep with presumed dreaming. When the same volunteers, however, were awakened from orthodox sleep over a similar length of time, no subsequent increase of sleep with rapid eye movements occurred.

So it was that in 1960 the idea was put about, often through the popular media, that you actually needed to dream and that if you did not get your dreams, you would later need to have extra dreams in compensation. Fisher and Dement wrote: 'The dream suppression procedure appeared to bring about a dream deficit – an increase in the pressure or need to dream. . . . During dream deprivation our subjects showed disturbances . . . tension and anxiety, difficulty in concentration, irritability . . . latent hallucinatory tendency. . . .' So it began to be said that if you did not dream you would go insane. While many other research workers have confirmed that if you are temporarily restricted in your paradoxical sleep you will catch up to some degree later, no one has found evidence that this will make anybody go insane, and the very idea could not have arisen nowadays when we know that dreaming occurs during any stage of sleep.

The new-born baby spends a very large part of its time in sleep with rapid eye movements, long before it could be said to have developed sufficient memories and understanding to construct a dream world. And if the antidepressant drugs known as mono-amine oxidase inhibitors are given to adults in sufficient quantity (they are the drugs that give bad headaches if cheese is eaten), then all signs of paradoxical sleep disappear and will remain absent for as many weeks or months as the drug continues to be taken. This certainly does not cause insanity; if anything the mental state improves.

We may still have psychological needs at night. After all, most of us would accept that we have psychological needs by day: we need to feel loved, needed, or admired. Many writers have thought that dreams in some way help the mind to sort out problems, to find solutions to personal problems of living, or to be creative in an artistic sense. The belief that dreams can serve a unique role in helping to understand the personality has become less popular than Freud would have wished, but the idea remains and some psycho-therapists will ask either individuals or groups of patients to recall recent dreams and then let the topics of recall serve for discussion to illustrate the problems of the daytime.

In summary, we can say that you can dream at any time of the night, though the richest dreaming is during paradoxical sleep. You can have daydreams too that do not differ sharply from nightdreams.

People who think they never dream are really people who forget (we all forget by far the greater part of our dreaming anyway).

Most people no longer believe in prophetic dreams, but dreams still form interesting talking points, whether for psychotherapy or for the amusement of your friends, and dreams will surely go on providing themes for creative writing, painting, music, and religious experience. We ourselves do not believe it matters whether you remember dreams or not, but if you do, then we hope that you enjoy them. Unfortunately, there are dreams that you have probably experienced at some time or other which are far from enjoyable.

# The two types of bad dream

The word 'nightmare' describes a dream in which some powerful force threatens to harm or destroy the sleeper. The word derives from the Sanskrit *mara*, or destroyer. Similarly, the French word for nightmare, *cauchemar*, comes from the same root, together with *caucher*, to tread upon. The root word *mara* became assimilated with the word 'mare' or female horse and much writing on the subject is linked with sexual symbolism, the horse often being seen as a symbol for powerful, active sexuality. It would however be wrong, in our opinion, to attribute all the violent feelings of a nightmare to sexual impulses, just as it would be foolish to attribute the horrors and violence of waking society to sexuality.

It is only modern research that has revealed the existence of two kinds of frightening dreams at night. There are the traditional nightmares, which are elaborate dreams coupled with paralysis and a feeling of inability to escape from the horror that is about to overwhelm you, and there are also night-terrors. The night-terrors are shorter and simpler dream experiences that occur during orthodox sleep, especially slow-wave sleep early in the night, whereas nightmares are really anxiety dreams that occur during paradoxical sleep – hence the feeling of paralysis – and are generally a feature of the later part of the night.

### Night-terrors
These are often immediately followed by sleep-walking, whereas the nightmares of paradoxical sleep are not. Both night-terrors and sleep-walking run in families and a tendency to both is almost certainly inherited. They occur especially during childhood and are less common among adults. They do not signify serious psychological

disturbance, any more than do occasional nightmares. However, like nightmares, night-terrors and sleep-walking do occur more frequently, if you are predisposed to them, when your waking life has lately become more anxious. An illustration of this is to be found in the battle-dreams of soldiers recently returned from the combat zone. The soldier may suddenly scream, rise from his bed and dive for shelter, shouting orders in his sleep.

Much commoner is the three-year-old who shrieks in the night, and sits up wide-eyed, as if shocked by some unknown horror. He may stumble out of bed, perhaps sobbing, and may need to be coaxed back by his distressed parents. By the age of four or five, such events are much less common. The child (or the adult) who has night-terrors, normally remembers nothing whatever of them. It is the parents who suffer the distress and they may be much in need of reassurance that time will bring alleviation, and that they need not fear that there is anything seriously amiss with their child. There are, of course, some children who continue to have night-terrors, or sleep-walk, into adolescence and adulthood. The events may be rare and become more frequent only when daytime stresses increase, such as when their mother or father goes to hospital, or when they start at a new school.

The night-terrors of adults have been investigated in New York by Dr Charles Fisher and his colleagues. They invited people who commonly experienced night-terrors to sleep in their laboratory, and then vigorously woke them up immediately after they began to cry out in their sleep. Mostly this occurred in the first couple of hours of sleep, and the mental experience described by those woken up was always simple, elemental terror, a feeling of being entrapped in a small area, of being left alone or abandoned, or of being about to be crushed or swallowed by a monster. There was a tremendous acceleration of the heart rate and a gasping for breath. Interestingly, the longer the deep orthodox sleep with EEG slow waves had just lasted, the more intense appeared to be the terror. There is no known way of avoiding night-terrors; but as they are usually forgotten on waking they are not a source of anxiety to those who experience them.

## Nightmares

These are instead protracted dream adventures, involving changing situations, which often feature people who persecute the dreamer. In story they are altogether more elaborate than the night-terrors. The nightmare could be called an anxiety dream.

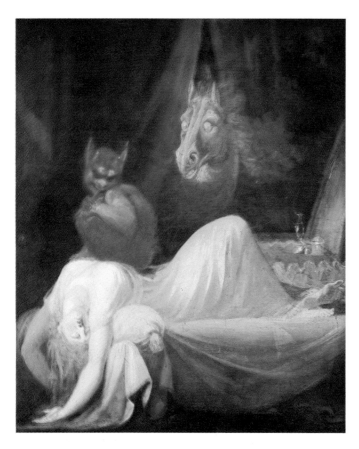

*The Nightmare* (1781) by Fuseli captures well the oppressive atmosphere of this type of bad dream. Compare with his picture on page 37.

Most of us have had a nightmare at some time in our lives, and many people have one every now and then; some people, though, are less fortunate. Those who have frequent nightmares often describe themselves as people with nervous trouble, or as having tension in the family, depression, loneliness or problems with alcohol.

In one London study, twenty women patients who were regarded by their family doctors as particularly anxious were asked to keep a note of all their dreams. The same twenty women were further classified into those who were very anxious and those who were only moderately anxious. The two sub-groups differed sharply in that the highly anxious patients reported having far more dreams in which people were aggressive or unfriendly towards them. If you are anxious or depressed and having nightmares unusually often, it would be sensible to try to tackle the underlying problems, perhaps with the help of your family doctor. Success may well be accompanied by a reduction in the frequency of your nightmares.

What about the belief that eating cheese before sleeping will cause

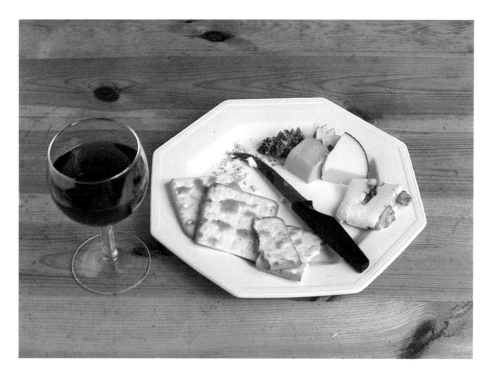

It's a popular misconception that eating cheese before bedtime causes nightmares. They are much more likely to result from drinking alcohol to excess.

nightmares? We are not convinced. Alcohol is a more important cause of nightmares than cheese. A drink in the afternoon or the evening may temporarily relieve daytime anxiety, but later on in the night there is a rebound, and bad dreams become more common as a consequence of the increased anxiety brought about by withdrawal of the alcohol, which is broken down in the body. As we shall be explaining in Chapter 7, coming off sleeping pills after a prolonged period of use will result in more nightmares and vivid dream experiences than usual.

# Sleep-walking and sleep-talking

The tendency to sleep-walk, as we have said, runs in families. The rising from bed may be entirely silent and peaceful, without any preceding night-terror, though often, and especially in children, there may be a general appearance of unhappiness.

Once again, the parents of the sleep-walking child need not fear some serious psychological abnormality; but if the child is especially anxious about some problem in daytime life, such as school exams, then the sleep-walking can be better understood and it can be more easily accepted that in time both the problem and the sleep-walking will go away.

In the meantime, though, it may be wise to take special precautions to avoid sharp obstructions, electric cables, or easily opened windows. Falling out of a window on a sleep-walk is in fact very unusual, but it is not uncommon for sleep-walkers to bruise themselves or draw blood by walking into things and perhaps bang their heads on sharp corners. We know by measuring their brain waves that sleep-walkers really are half-asleep. Their powers of discrimination and efficient control of where they are walking are lower than during full wakefulness. They will not remember their nocturnal excursions, unless thoroughly awakened by other people, or by the cold when wandering outside the house. Commonly an episode of sleep-walking involves the act of urination, not always directed into the conventional receptacle.

Apart from daytime anxiety, causes of more frequent sleep-walking include alcohol intake, and a whole variety of drugs that act upon the nervous system, or, even more potently, a combination of some drug (a pain-killer, for example) and alcohol.

One man who has been to our sleep laboratory, a lawyer, used to sleep-walk often when he had drunk too much vodka. He told us that if he were away from home and staying in a hotel, he would take care at night to hide the key to his room in elaborate fashion, so as not to be able to find it when sleep-walking, having earlier once found himself wandering away from the hotel in the middle of the night. On another occasion he caused considerable embarrassment by ending a sleep-walk in the bed of a then unoccupied room, and alarming a lady guest who arrived at a subsequent hour.

Sleep-talking of a vigorous kind seems to run in the same families as those who sleep-walk; and often the sleep-walker will sleep-talk at the same time. But, of course, we can all of us sleep-talk on occasions. It is a time for talking gibberish rather than for betraying closely kept secrets. Sleep-talking occurs at any time of night. It need not give cause for concern, though it may well elicit amusement from a bed-partner – and may cause the listener a few minutes lost sleep. Most other causes of lost sleep are, unfortunately, less entertaining.

# 5. SLEEP LOSS AND WAYS TO REDUCE IT

## Common causes of lost sleep

We all lose sleep from time to time, and no one ever likes to do so. For most of us it is a rare event to lose an entire night's sleep; it may happen perhaps when a baby is born in the middle of the night, or when we make an intercontinental flight. Then, next night, we sleep long and heavily, though it usually takes another two nights to feel really back to normal.

Much commoner is a partial loss of a night's sleep. Again it may be a consequence of our activities: travel, possibly, or a social gathering. The gathering may be a hectic occasion, but not necessarily a worrying one. Most of us expect to lose sleep from time to time for one of these reasons. What none of us likes is to be awake most of the night because of a sudden new worry or personal problem in life. There can be few things as frustrating as when some unexpected anxiety keeps you fitfully tossing and turning on a night when you feel you really need a good night's sleep to face the day ahead. Equally disconcerting is waking in the small hours and finding yourself beginning to turn daytime problems over in your mind. Before you know it, you feel wide awake, and anxiety about not being able to get back to sleep only makes things worse. The presence of a peacefully sleeping partner may well make you feel even more acutely conscious of being awake.

At the end of this chapter we shall be giving you some suggestions for getting to sleep, and keeping your loss of sleep to a minimum, but more than likely your problem may rapidly resolve itself and you will soon have the opportunity to catch up on what sleep was lost. It is reassuring to know that catching up on sleep after accumulating an 'overdraft' seems to be a fact of life. In one research study, diaries of hours of sleep kept by students showed that many of them worked or played late into the night and yet had to get up early in the morning on weekdays, but that at week-ends they were able to catch up by sleeping some fourteen hours at a stretch.

## Babies and young children

For many of you partial loss of a night's sleep is a recurrent burden, almost the routine for years. If you are the mother of a small baby, and have slightly older children who may also demand attention in the night, you may know what it is to feel that you never get enough sleep.

The problem arises because of the immaturity of a new-born baby's biological clock, the baby's lack of social conditioning, and, of course, its need for frequent and regular feeding. Over many millions of years we evolved in a world in which light and dark came and went every twenty-four hours and even in the new-born baby there is a circadian rhythm (see Chapter 1) that makes it fall asleep more easily at some times of the twenty-four hours than at others. However, the times when it wakes and sleeps are more determined by the shorter ultradian rhythm, which in the baby does not occur in 100-minute cycles, as in adults, but in roughly 50-minute ones. The baby sleeps, and then after two, three or four multiples of 50 minutes, it wakes and yells for food. If it does so by day when its parents are up and about, it is likely to receive a lot more social stimulation than if it wakes in the night. Under the influence of these social pressures the infant soon learns to conform to the same 24-hour pattern as the adults around it and to do most of its sleeping at night.

As at any age, there are big individual differences in the total duration of sleep, but the average baby takes about 14 hours of sleep out of the 24 hours in its first weeks of life, but after a year or two this has reduced to 10–12 hours. Babies will take for themselves the amount of sleep they need, and since some babies need less than others, it is inevitable that quite a lot of young couples will think that their particular baby is the world's worst sleeper, because it only wants about 8 or 9 hours, or even less.

However little sleep your baby needs, there are things you can try in order to cut down both the time it is awake at night and your own sleep loss to a minimum, although it's often the case that nothing you do will make any difference to how much your baby sleeps. Most wakeful babies are just inherently short sleepers, so there's no need to feel guilty or inadequate as a parent if all your efforts go unrewarded. Many parents, however, find that attending promptly to their baby's persistent crying, even if it is not due for a feed, makes the baby quicker to settle, and so reduces the time they spend awake.

Nowadays babies are often put in separate rooms. To be alone and in the dark can awaken primitive fears, which are more likely to

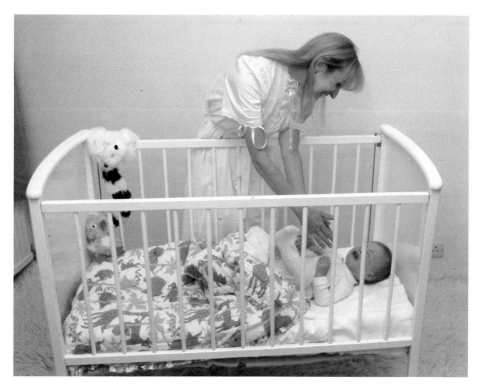

Wakeful babies are a common cause of lost sleep for parents. Many babies simply need less sleep than average.

make an infant cry and demand the attention of its parents. This does not mean a child is in need of disciplining, though if the baby is always rewarded by being taken into the parental bed whenever it cries at night, it may eventually learn to cry in order to achieve the invariable reward. Babies, though, need cuddles and security rather than a disciplinary code. It is up to you to work out a routine that suits you and your baby. Careful juggling of feeding times, perhaps so the baby is fed at the time you go to bed rather than two hours later, can also cut down the amount of time you are up during the night.

A warm, loved and well-fed baby in a clean nappy or diaper usually sleeps well between feeds, but all mothers and fathers can expect to have the occasional bad night. If left to cope alone with the baby, the effect of several bad nights in a row can make mothers irritable (as we shall be discussing later in the chapter). At times like these the father's support is especially important. He can help to bring things back to normal by taking on night duty for a few nights

– over the weekend, perhaps – thus giving the mother a chance to catch up on her sleep.

It is not just babies that cause parents to lose sleep; it can be older children as well. A doctor in Edinburgh, Dr Ronald Seiler, asked the parents of 250 children aged under six years, all in his local practice, whether their child was or had been a sleep problem to them on account of wakefulness, restlessness or night fears. No less than 40 per cent of parents regarded their children as having caused them sleep problems, which means that children's sleep that brings about worry and exhaustion for the parents is so common as to be well within the range of normal. The comforting thing that Dr Seiler discovered was that, once past the fourth birthday, most children ceased to cause problems for their parents during the night. Hope on the horizon for most parents of small infants! Even more parents can look forward to those times when, in late adolescence, it will be difficult to get their offspring to wake up.

### Being 'on call'
Junior hospital doctors work long hours, are often 'on call' for most of their supposed rest time, and liable to have to get out of bed more than once in the middle of any night. Many too feel an intense sense of responsibility for their sick patients that drives them to visit the wards when they might be having a little time off.

### Long-term causes
Yet other people suffer worries and adversities that are sustained, and that do not go away, over periods of many months or even years. The sources of worry may be in their environment, or within themselves, perhaps arising from a period of mental ill-health. We will be considering their long-term sleep problems, and others, which have a more specific physical cause, in the next chapter, Insomnia.

# How sleep loss will affect you

What are the effects of long-continued reduction in the usual amount of sleep? It depends very much on how stressful is the cause of the reduction of sleep, and, of course, by just how much the sleep is reduced. In San Diego, California, experiments were carried out with volunteer couples who, over a period of months, gradually cut down their sleep duration from about seven hours nightly to about five hours, on a regular basis, and without any striking impairment of their mental or physical efficiency. However, they could not escape from the feeling of fatigue, and were unable to reduce their nocturnal sleep to a shorter period.

Research into the psychological problems faced by young hospital doctors has been carried out both in Cambridge, England, and in New York. In Cambridge a variety of efficiency tests showed that the doctors' professional performance was quite frequently impaired because of their hours of work; and, most particularly, it was found that they were unpredictable in their efficiency, sometimes doing as well as their natural best, and at other times being very inefficient indeed. Many of the doctors themselves felt under stress and, for example, felt particular difficulty in getting to sleep after a middle-of-the-night telephone conversation about a sick patient. They felt anxious about their sicker patients and had nightmares when they did sleep.

In New York the doctors' loss of sleep had similar effects. Some had lapses of memory: 'I would forget what I had just said so that my next sentence would make no sense.' Many described becoming irritable: 'If you're on two nights in a row, you want to do as little as possible. You give bad care. I am irritated all the time then; I can only think of one thing at a time. I can't react to complexity. I give bad care to my patients, unfortunately. When I am tired, I don't give a goddamn.' Another described how: 'The fatigue is a stress that gets me depressed. The nurses kid me that I crawl into a corner when I am tired. I become a monster then and I know it. On the last ward the nurses were inexperienced and bothered me all the time. I am ashamed of how nasty I was. I had no patience.' How many mothers of young children could echo words like these!

The sudden loss of reasonableness, the snapping and shouting and the later feelings of shame are not the kind of things that can be measured in laboratory research, but they are very important consequences of long-continued reduction in the hours of sleep. It is for reasons like these that there are rules and regulations that limit the length of tiring duties for some classes of occupation, like long-distance truck-driving, or for aircrew. But such rules never apply to the mothers of small children, nor to business people and statesmen and women who fly around the world having conferences, often working till late into the night and then getting up early, with their biological clocks badly disturbed by long-distance travel. One must suppose that many of them are much worse impaired in their judgements than they themselves would realize, and feelings of irritability can hardly be ideal for coming to decisions that affect the destinies

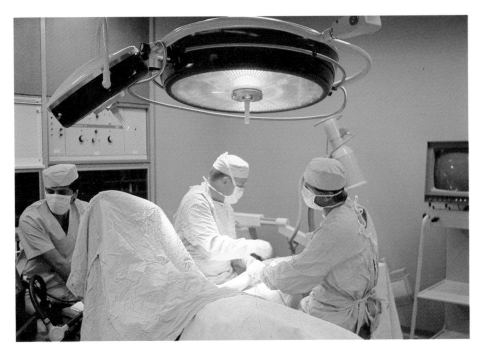

Young hospital doctors regularly lose sleep in the course of their work. Research has shown that irritability and impaired judgement are the most common effects of continued sleep loss.

of huge multinational companies, and indeed of whole nations.

Are people who feel that they are just poor sleepers, never getting a good night's rest – even though there is no easily identifiable cause – liable to suffer in the same way? We cannot give a definite answer. If they feel depressed and irritable by day, it cannot with certainty be attributed to a bad night, for it may be more a matter of individual temperament, that also causes them to sleep badly. We ourselves have sympathy with the view that such people are partly depressed and irritable because of bad sleep, and not just because they have a constitution that makes them both irritable and sleepless.

## You will sleep if you really need to

Anxiety about sleep loss is itself a common cause of lost sleep. So to find out more about the effects of losing sleep we have kept volunteers awake day and night. After about seventy-two hours of continuous lack of sleep they start seeing things that are not there, their co-operation begins to flag, they may become suspicious and even do and say strange things. The one thing they all have in common is that they fall asleep whenever they have a moment undisturbed, even walking along the street. The lesson to learn from this is that when we are short of sleep, Nature takes care to look after our interests, and if we really need sleep, and have, take or are given the opportunity to sleep, then we can rely on Nature to give us rest.

We have already described in this chapter some of the unpleasant consequences of lost sleep, irritability, for example; but we must emphasize that you cannot die of loss of sleep, nor will you suffer long-term mental or physical ill-effects as a result. You can take comfort from the fact that sleep is a self-regulating system so that when we really need it, we get it and almost nothing will stop us.

Before we leave the subject of the impairments in how people feel and act after loss of sleep, we ought to mention the opposite side of the coin as revealed by the research of Drs Taub and Berger in Santa Cruz, California. They have shown very clearly that sleeping longer than usual, or sleeping at irregular times, can lead to just about the same kinds of inefficiencies, feelings of low spirits and irritability, as can be brought about by lack of sleep.

# Keeping your sleep loss to a minimum

Some books claim to have the definitive answer to everyone's problem of getting to sleep: 'Use the positive thought-control method', 'Learn self-management', 'Take up transcendental meditation', 'Relax yourself to sleep on a water bed', 'Try hypnotic sleep therapy'. All easy advice to give, but we believe that while a mind at peace is the most important prerequisite for sleep there is no simple knack that can achieve this ideal state.

There are several things, though, you can try that may help you to get to sleep; although what is successful for one person, might not be for another. Again, it is really up to you to find out by trial and error what works best for you. On the other hand there are things we would advise you to avoid that are bound to cause you to lose more sleep than perhaps you do already, and we will be dealing with these at the end of the chapter.

**What you can do during the day**

**Getting up early in the morning**   As we explained in Chapter 1, this is probably your surest way of falling asleep quickly at night. Try getting up earlier as a matter of routine; the more regular you are in your habits, the better will be the quality of your sleep.

**Exercise** Most people in our modern society, especially in middle age, take far too little exercise. Many of us have had the experience of taking a good walk in the morning, and then falling asleep after lunch, or of having a long walk in the afternoon and wanting to drop off to sleep earlier than usual in the evening.

Very severe, unaccustomed exercise, though, will disturb sleep, for the heart keeps on beating fast, the temperature stays raised and the whole body remains in an overheated and excited state through the night. Strenuous exercise too close to bedtime will have similar effects.

It is known that if fit people take exercise on one day and not on another, they tend to fall asleep more quickly after the exercise and sleep rather longer on that night than the other; and in the case of athletes, at least, there is rather more of the slow-wave sleep, the really deep sleep, after exercise. At Edinburgh we also found that extra growth hormone was released into the blood during sleep, to help the tissues restore themselves after the extra exercise by day. So more exercise means better sleep, but what again is important is regularity of habits, and sudden gross excesses should be avoided. Indeed, if you plan to take up a strenuous form of exercise (jogging or tennis, for example) or to return to a sport after a long layoff, take it easy at first – especially if you are over forty. There is no reason why you cannot achieve a reasonable degree of fitness at any age, but the older you are, the more gradual you must be.

### Pre-sleep routines

Before going to bed try to direct your attention away from the pressures of the day. Some find practising a hobby a good way of winding down in the evening; others prefer to watch television (obviously it makes sense not to watch the late-night horror film if the macabre disturbs you); and for many, a hot bath helps relaxation. This is a time to avoid, if you can, emotional arguments, excitement and intense mental or physical activity (apart from sex), as the more alert and stimulated you are, the longer it will take you to fall asleep.

Once in bed you will tend to succumb to sleep more quickly if you are relaxed and warm, and if your basic needs for food and sex are satisfied. Your bedtime reading matter is your own choice, but a long romantic novel may well have you nodding off faster than a racy thriller. During the cold winter months ensure that your bedroom is warmed up before you go to bed, and that you have sufficient

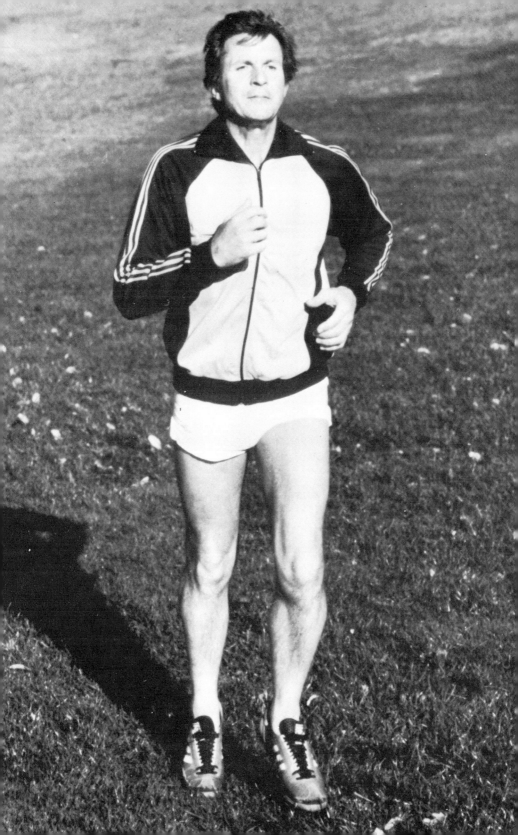

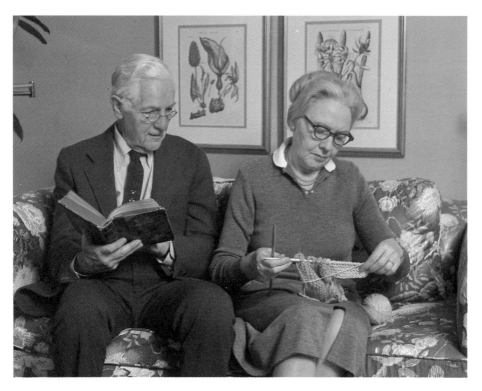

Relaxing in the evening is a good way to prepare for sleep.

nightwear and bedclothes to prevent you from waking up shivering in the small hours.

Although, as we have said, we don't believe there is any foolproof sleep-inducing technique, we do think that it is possible to have some degree of control over your thoughts as you close your eyes and prepare to drop off. Try deliberately to direct your mind away from troubling, stressful and unhappy thoughts, and don't start attempting to solve problems that have been worrying you during the day. Put them away for tomorrow, let go and relax. Picturing some pleasant scenario – a summer vacation perhaps – may well lead you on to tranquil trains of thought more suited to sleep. Banishing daytime worries from your mind is just as important if you wake in the middle of the night. This is when time spent awake probably causes most concern about loss of sleep. But there is no need to be weighed down by this added anxiety, for as we said earlier, loss of sleep will do you no harm, and in the long run you will get the sleep you need.

We realize that for the seriously depressed person lying awake, it may be impossible to stop worrying. But other people find what suits them. One seventy-year-old man told us he had cured his sleep problem by getting out of bed at about one o'clock every morning and then taking an ice-cold bath, after which he returned to bed and slept. Many people, after lying awake, do get up, pass urine, walk about or drink tea. Do what comes naturally, by all means, but as a general rule regularity is the thing to aim for. Daytime is the time for being up and about, night-time for lying in bed and not for constantly trotting around.

Most people like to curl up on their sides or tummies, rather than lie on their backs for going to sleep, but they will spend much of the later night on their backs. It is best to find a really comfortable position as soon as possible, because the more restless you are – the more tossing and turning you do – the more delayed you will be in falling asleep.

If you want to get to sleep quickly, it helps to find a really comfortable position. Many people like to curl up on their sides like this.

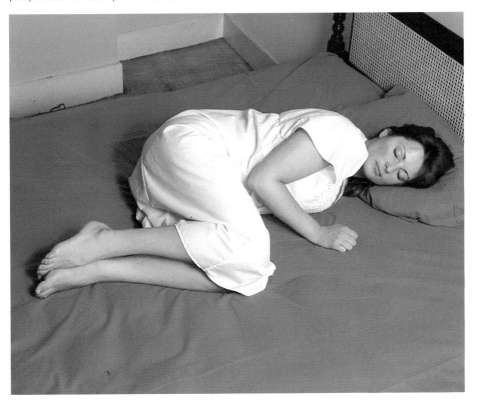

## The bedroom

You make your choice over the colour of the wallpaper, it matters only to you, and you decide for yourself whether you want to leave the door open and have the dog thumping his tail on the floor in the middle of the night, or the cat to jump on top of you. If the summer sun shines into your eyes in the morning, turn the bed around or put up thicker curtains or drapes. And whether you sleep with the window open or closed is again purely a matter of taste – and warmth. There is no evidence that fresh air is better for sleep than stale air, or vice versa; but do keep warm, especially if you have chest trouble.

**Beds**  If your bed is making sleep more difficult for you, because it is old and lumpy, perhaps, or because it sags and forces you and your partner both to roll down to the dip in the centre of the bed and to fight in your sleep to clamber up again, it is well worth considering buying a new bed. Some people will buy a new lounge suite to impress the neighbours, but carry on with the same ancient bed and worn-out mattress, which might be preventing them from getting a proper night's rest.

A good bed has a sprung-base to match a spring mattress and it should not sag. The degree of firmness you require depends partly on your weight and partly on your own preference. The mattress should be firm enough to support your back when, during paradox-

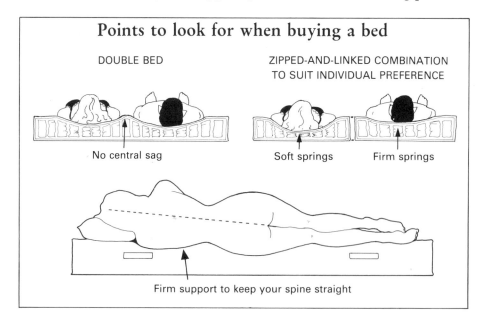

## Points to look for when buying a bed

DOUBLE BED

ZIPPED-AND-LINKED COMBINATION
TO SUIT INDIVIDUAL PREFERENCE

No central sag

Soft springs

Firm springs

Firm support to keep your spine straight

ical sleep, all the muscles go limp and throw the load on the ligaments. Our ancestors slept on the floor of their caves and so our bodies have been designed for sleeping on firm surfaces. It takes time, after your old sagger, to get used to a new bed and mattress, so give it a few weeks, and in time it will prove itself. Pillows should not be too deep and should be soft so as to be gentler on the ears.

If you are disturbed by your partner's movements on a double mattress, try sleeping on two single beds zipped and linked together. This has the added advantage of allowing each partner to have the type of mattress he or she prefers.

**Gadgets**  Rabbit's foot charms have no action on sleep and the only bedroom gadget that has a genuine effect is a box sold in some countries for producing monotonous beating sounds, like heartbeats, or the sound of waves on the sea shore. Monotonous noises really do induce sleep a bit more quickly, but no one knows if the effectiveness will persist over weeks and months.

## Sleeping drugs and alcohol
There is a popular misconception that a tot of spirits at bedtime is the surest guarantee of a good night's sleep. But we are convinced that using alcohol to help you get to sleep is definitely a bad idea, especially if you are depressed, irritable and tired.

Alcohol does send you to sleep more quickly, but it will disturb your sleep later on in the night. We would also advise you not to turn to sleeping pills as a long-term solution to your sleeping problem. However, reasonable compromises have to be found to suit every individual situation. Taking a prescribed sleeping drug on one or two nights consecutively can be a boon to some people, without the risk of them experiencing bad sleep afterwards.

Hospitals are noisy and frightening places and if you have to go in for an operation, you will probably have trouble sleeping. On such an occasion it seems eminently reasonable that you should have a sleeping drug on the few nights before your operation, though care should be taken that regular intake does not develop and that the drug is stopped by the time you return home. Crises just as worrying as an operation can occur within the home. Here the same commonsense use of drugs should again apply, but only as a rare prop.

You will discover in Chapter 7 that we are not overenthusiastic about sleeping drugs, but at least the ones that are prescribed and are taken in carefully measured doses are both cheaper and also much less damaging to the liver and the nervous system than alcohol.

# 6. INSOMNIA

## Long-term dissatisfaction with your sleep

Insomnia is a very common problem: around 15 per cent of all patients attending their family doctor complain of it (often as one of a number of complaints). In the last chapter we dealt specifically with sleep loss, and in many people's minds this is equated with insomnia. But insomnia is not simply a matter of losing sleep. In fact, as we shall be showing at the end of this chapter, the vast majority of insomniacs actually lose far less sleep than they feel they do. We hope this will be reassuring to all those who experience long-term dissatisfaction with their sleep – for this is what insomnia really is. When someone says he suffers from insomnia he is saying something about his subjective experience: that he feels his sleep is displeasing to him because it is either slow in coming, broken by periods of wakefulness or because it leaves him feeling tired and unrefreshed by day.

Insomnia is not a disease, it is a complaint, much as a pain in the tummy is not a disease but a complaint. Like a tummy pain, insomnia can be the result of any one of several different root causes. And, like the complaint of pain, insomnia takes on a social dimension by evoking a direct response from other people. The insomniac, no less than the sufferer from physical pain, wants the sympathy and support of close family and friends – and, when the dissatisfaction becomes intolerable, the family doctor.

Our subjective experiences cannot be measured by someone else, but only by each of us 'measuring' our pain today on some sort of inner scale and telling either ourselves, or somebody else, that it is worse than yesterday, or not nearly as bad as it was a week ago. Nor can we say if our pain is worse than another's. Similarly, we cannot say if one person's subjective experience of poor sleep indicates a greater degree of poorness than that described by another person. There may be no difference at all in the amount of disruption of sleep and no difference in its restorative quality (though we are not yet able to measure this last very accurately). It is just that some people can be more affected by the feeling of bad sleep than others.

# Who tends to suffer from insomnia?

The emotions, of course, are inextricably tied to the way we feel we sleep, and the way we describe it. Drs McGhie and Russell carried out a survey at Glasgow and Dundee in Scotland of 2,500 people of varying age and social class, and found that those who thought they were of a nervous temperament were also more often those who felt that they slept badly.

Your physical characteristics can also influence the way you sleep. As we will be discussing in more detail in Chapter 8, people who are underweight, or losing weight, may find they experience poor sleep.

**More women than men**

In many countries of the world, surveys have been conducted in which large numbers of people have been asked to say how many hours of sleep they think they get; how lightly or deeply they think they sleep; whether they waken frequently in the night; or whether they think either they have difficulty in getting to sleep, or wake up early in the morning, or just do not feel refreshed by their sleep. The results of the surveys show that around twice as many women report problems with their sleep as men, and this is true for all age groups.

Despite the fact that no one has been able to prove there is an objective difference between the sleep of men and women, one possible explanation may be that as most women do not expend as much energy by day as men, they may not wear out their body tissues so much by day, and so Nature may have designed them to need less intensely restorative sleep at night. In other words, women may genuinely have less need of sound sleep than men, in the same way as they need a smaller daily energy intake in the form of food and drink. Another possible reason is that women's restorative sleep is in some way disturbed by the constant change in their hormonal pattern during the menstrual cycle. We cannot at the present say for sure why women suffer from insomnia more than men; clearly a great deal more research is needed in this area.

**The menopause** Many women pass through later middle life without being troubled by the traditional symptoms of the menopause or change of life. Others, and especially if the menopause occurs earlier than average, are burdened by unpleasant hot flushes, feelings of depression, irritability towards those around them, and by a sense of poor and broken sleep. Some seek to alleviate these feelings with alcohol, many with pills for their nerves, or with sleeping drugs, which in the long run have a detrimental effect on their sleep that can persist even when the menopause has become a thing of the past. Some doctors believe it is possible to relieve the unpleasant symptoms of the menopause – including insomnia – by prescribing pills containing the hormone oestrogen.

To test how well this treatment works, we invited thirty-two menopausal women who were dissatisfied with their sleep to come to our laboratory for several months at a stretch so that we could monitor their sleep by measuring their electrical brain waves. We gave all the volunteers identical-looking pills to take, without telling them which contained only an inactive substance, and which contained oestrogen. Over the weeks there were many improvements in how the women felt and slept, but the degree of improvement in sleep was greater among those who were taking the genuine oestrogen pills than among those who took the inactive ones.

This so-called 'hormone replacement therapy' for women after the menopause will also prevent the thinning of the bones that occurs throughout the rest of their lives, as well as having the small but definite beneficial effect on their sleep. How wise it is to interfere with the natural course of ageing in this way remains a subject of much debate among doctors, and the history of medical treatments should make us cautious, in case in future decades we learn that the treatment can have unforeseen disadvantages.

## The elderly

As people approach old age dissatisfaction with their sleep tends to become more common; and this is reflected in the increased rate of prescriptions for sleeping pills from their doctors, again, especially among women. In the Scottish survey mentioned previously, nearly 45 per cent of 75-year-old women regularly took drugs for sleep.

Contact with other people is very important for older people, whether with family or friends or through social clubs and organizations. Outside interests and support may well provide the psychological uplift needed to restore a greater degree of satisfaction with sleep.

Whether we feel we are ageing gracefully or not, our brains are slowly losing tissue – at the rate of about 2 g per year – from as early as the age of thirty. We must stress that there is plenty of reserve tissue in the brain, but with time the effects of age must inevitably tell on any of us. As the brain changes with age, so its demand for blood is reduced, hand in hand with a slight lessening of powers of concentration and memory (happily often compensated for by a greater degree of carefulness and conscientiousness). The greater disruption of sleep marches in step with these other brain changes. The actual duration of sleep may not alter much, but the consolidation of night-time sleep into an almost unbroken stretch happens less frequently and less effectively.

In Gainesville, Florida, a group of research workers used electrical brain wave recordings to study the sleep of healthy male and female volunteers of differing ages, ranging from infancy to their seventies. They made measurements of how frequently sleep was broken spontaneously during the night, and were able to confirm that as age advances, so sleep does indeed become more broken for both men and women. Many elderly people feel they can compensate by taking daytime naps; and so it is that the child's pattern of a nap in the early afternoon often returns with old age.

## Young people

We should not allow our emphasis on age as an accompaniment of dissatisfaction with sleep to blind us to the fact that there are a number of children, adolescents and young adults who feel there is something wrong with their sleep. In Drs McGhie and Russell's survey of 2,500 people in Scotland, there were 400 persons aged 15–24 years and among these there were 5 per cent who regarded their sleep as disturbed and who often took pills, whether prescribed drugs or remedies bought from pharmacies. In a similar study of 1,600 people in Gainesville, Florida, 6 per cent of the 18–19 year olds said that they found it difficult to sleep.

Like their elders, young people who feel troubled by their sleep are also those who feel troubled by their nerves. In one study in Chicago, Dr Monroe selected from among 200 students a group of 16 who considered themselves particularly poor sleepers and a similar group of 16 especially good sleepers. In their answers to questionnaires and in the assessment of their personality, the poor sleepers appeared to have a more depressed outlook on life.

On the other side of the world, in Melbourne, Australia, a very similar study was carried out by Dr M. Johns on medical students of average age 21, and once again complaints of poor sleep and nightmares were associated with psychological problems, and especially with a sense of low self-esteem.

There was a further, more detailed and revealing study in a senior high school in the San Francisco Bay area. Among 639 pupils, 12 per cent said that they thought they had persistent sleep problems, such as taking more than 45 minutes to fall asleep at least three times a week, and waking up during the night for 30 minutes or more at least three times a week. These pupils were distinguished from the others by the worry and tension revealed in their answers to the other questions. They described more personal and family problems than their class-mates. They particularly mentioned low self-esteem, and feeling moody and depressed most of the time. This suggests that, as with adults, insomnia goes hand in hand with psychological problems by day.

It is not merely a matter of having only a small number of hours sleep, for in that same high school the pupils made estimates of how many hours they slept, and there were 23 who said that they usually only slept for 3 to 5 hours, and while 12 of these pupils were among those who regarded themselves as poor sleepers, the other 11 had no complaints at all about their sleep. It is not duration of sleep, but the sense of satisfaction with sleep that counts. Here once again is this link between contentment with nocturnal sleep and general psychological contentment by day.

# Identifiable causes of insomnia and ways to cope with them

### Anxiety and depression

When special anxieties come into our lives, we tend to have especially broken sleep, with worries coming thick and fast during the night. A feeling of depression in spirits or mood is a normal experience after disappointments – being made redundant, for example – or after bereavements, or if we are waiting with a sense of foreboding for something to happen that we know will be unpleasant, such as an appearance in court on account of drunken driving, or in connection with a divorce. Indeed, sometimes the sense of waiting with uncertainty is worse than the final knowledge of the outcome. Depression under these circumstances is an understandable reaction to the circumstances of life, and it will often be accompanied by sleep that really is impaired.

To talk to others about your bereavement is not a sign of weakness. It helps you to adjust to the new pattern of life. If some other stress affecting sleep arises from a situation over which you have control, try to resolve it by decision-making, and the sooner the better. Two years of bitter litigation can do you harm: better to settle by negotiation for something less and get the affair over in two months. Better when suffering anxiety to be driven to a decision for action than to take tranquillizers and then be forever putting off the resolution of life's difficulties.

So many hurts arise from family relationships; and it is up to someone to say sorry first, perhaps again and again. To kiss and make up at bedtime is better than resentfully lying there half-awake. When the time of stress has passed, the depression can be expected to lift and sleep return to normal.

If anxieties cause bad night after bad night and you feel that soon you may no longer be able to cope, a change in life-style – either temporary or more permanent – may be the only solution. A vacation might be all that's required to get back to a more relaxed pattern of sleeping and give back the energy you need to deal with the problems at work or at home. If, though, you find it impossible to shrug off the anxieties wherever you are, and your sleep troubles seem to be locked into an ever-worsening spiral, then maybe the time has come to tackle the underlying causes by making a radical alteration to the way you live: changing jobs, perhaps, or taking a position with less pressure and responsibility.

There are, however, some people for whom sustained lowering of spirits and a sense of inner anxiety and foreboding cannot be explained or understood in terms of life's circumstances; and we recognize that they are suffering from an illness affecting the nervous system. Their usual energies and interests desert them; they no longer feel able to cope with the simple tasks of life; their concentration seems impaired; they become self-critical and feel that they should 'fight it' or pull themselves together. They often say they are feeling weepy, more sensitive about what other people might be thinking of them, and sometimes that life is not worth going on with – and all this in someone who has generally been a lively and active person and for whom there are no special problems manifest in life at the time.

The gloomy thoughts often revolve around awareness of the body, with fears of cancer or of going out of the mind near to hand; and never more so than in the small hours of the morning, for it is then that such people feel especially wakeful. They probably do not wake up more during the night than many others of their own age, but the thoughts that come are not happy and will sometimes lead them to pace about in the night, make tea and sit in the kitchen, worrying. Depression of this kind is one of the most important causes of the complaint of insomnia that doctors seek to recognize, because there are treatments available for this illness – usually antidepressant drugs. When the general depression is relieved, sleep recovers too.

A depressive illness is one of the most common kinds of psychiatric trouble, probably affecting at least 10 per cent of the population one or more times in life. So-called postnatal depression can be severe in a small proportion of women after childbirth. Depressive illness can affect anyone at any age, but it is more likely to occur for the first time in the latter half of life. For an unlucky few there may be repeated episodes, and some can be troubled by what is termed manic-depressive illness. Their periods of depression are set against spells of weeks at a time when they feel excessively energetic, confident and happy. They have a zest, perhaps, for rising at three in the morning to rush around singing and whistling while doing the housework, their elation reaching a pitch that other people recognize as unnatural. Fortunately, this condition responds well to modern treatments, once the first feelings of reluctance about seeking help are overcome.

Inevitably, depressive illnesses sometimes occur at a time of life when there are also genuine problems surrounding the sufferer, so that the recognition of whether or not the poor sleep and depression are caused by something to be regarded as an illness, and treated as such, is not always quite as easy as it has been made to sound here. It is a matter for your family doctor to decide, and, if he or she wishes, a psychiatrist too.

## Recurrent noise

The link we have already noted between satisfaction or dissatisfaction with sleep on the one hand, and the sense of contentment on the other, emerges when people complain of being kept awake by noise.

People who live near airports, for example, are subjected to noise, to which many of them very reasonably object. Interviewers called upon nearly 6,000 people living near London Airport, the districts in which they lived being graded into areas of particularly high aircraft noise, and areas of lesser aircraft noise. The interviewers asked questions about health, difficulty in getting to sleep at night, waking frequently in the night, and also asked about the degree to which each person felt annoyed by the amount of aircraft noise.

Overall, those who lived in areas subject to high levels of aircraft noise, did seem to suffer some impairment to their psychological

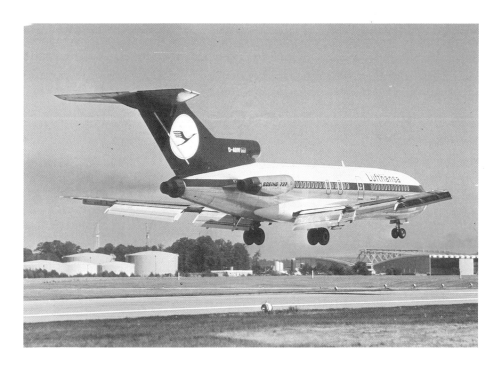

health and particularly complained of difficulty in getting to sleep and of waking in the night. Much the most striking association, though, was between a declaration of feeling annoyed by aircraft noise and complaints about difficulty in sleeping. We can get used to regular noises, and sleep through them, but if they are noises about which we hold angry opinions, then sure enough they will keep us awake.

Widely spaced double-glazing helps to keep out noise, and some find ear-plugs helpful, although most people don't persist with them. Most important, if there is nothing you can do to stop the noise, is to try to forgive the rudenesses offered by its originators.

## Physical discomfort

**Pain** Severe toothache will keep us awake on occasions, and a recommended dose of a mild pain-killer such as aspirin or paracetamol (acetaminophen in the United States) will usually reduce the level of pain so that we can sleep through the night and awake next morning ready for a visit to the dentist. It is worth checking the contents of proprietary across-the-counter pain-killers, as many contain caffeine, which is a stimulant that makes sleep harder to attain.

Pain at night can be a problem for those who suffer from arthritis.

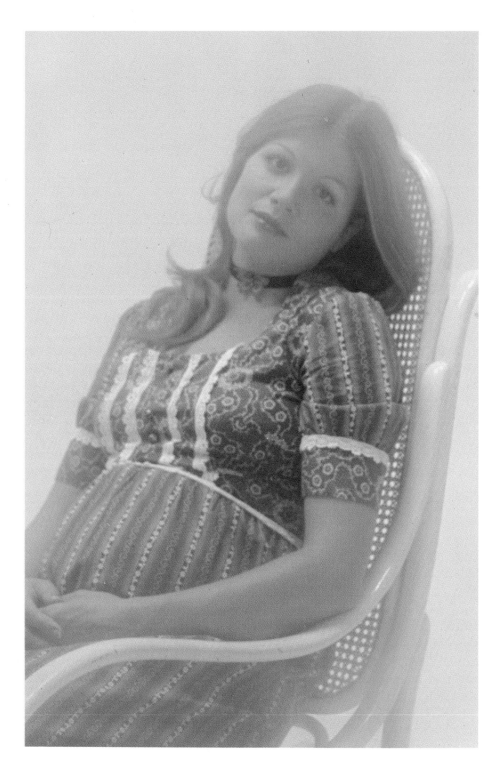

They get stiff in their joints when they lie still, so that when they move they experience a sudden twinge of pain which briefly disturbs their sleep. While generally it is true that too many people take too many pain-killers, we would advise you, if your sleep is persistently broken by pain to take a pain-killer prescribed by your family doctor rather than to court sounder sleep with sleeping pills. If you suffer regularly from chronic back pain, then a good bed is essential. It should have a firm base and mattress.

**Threadworms**   Children more often than adults get threadworms, which have a curious biological clock of their own that prompts them to wriggle out just at bedtime. Sleep delayed by an itchy anus should prompt suspicion of threadworms, inspection of the anus and faeces, and, if the worms are visible as white, 2-cm/1-in long threads, a visit to the doctor.

## Pregnancy

Expectant mothers in the last few months of pregnancy are likely to be feeling tired; and when they want to get as much sleep as possible to cope with the impending labour, they may find it more difficult to sleep. The enlarged abdomen makes it difficult to lie comfortably; the baby's kicking prevents a consolidated night's rest; and they may need to urinate several times during the night. In addition to these problems, they may be anxious about the delivery, the baby's health or even whether a particular sleeping position might harm the foetus.

First of all, let us say there is no position you can adopt while you are asleep that will affect the baby. Of our suggestions for better sleep in the previous chapter, probably the best for the sleep and health of pregnant women is a little regular daily exercise: a good walk in the fresh air is all you need. Pregnancy is a time when back-ache is especially common, and a firm mattress to support the ligaments while you sleep is again sensible.

We would advise expectant mothers not to take sleeping drugs, because the unborn child could be affected by any drugs the mother takes. They can cross the placental barrier and with some drugs there is a small risk of malformations of the foetus (alcohol is no exception). Doctors prescribe as few drugs as possible during pregnancy, and use only those they know are safest. Although there are mild sedatives, it is better to avoid the possible sense of guilt that might follow should anything at all happen to be wrong with the baby when it is born, whether the abnormality could have been caused by the drug or not.

## Breathing difficulties

People who have heart and chest diseases, and difficulty in breathing at night, also often suffer from broken sleep, though the extent to which they feel it is a disability is rarely expressed in such vivid terms of dissatisfaction as by many a person sound in heart and lung, but of a tense, anxious disposition.

**Bronchitis and wheezing**  A warm atmosphere is good to sleep in for most people with chronic bronchitis. In cold climates, the heating of winter air also means a very dry atmosphere, and, for children or adults with wheezy chests, warm but more humid air is advisable. The old-fashioned steam kettle in the bedroom achieved this. A modern kettle is just as effective, as can be more expensive humidification systems; but if a dry, hacking cough is ruining your sleep, one or two wet towels hung in the room – perhaps on a warm radiator – can at least help, and many find comfort from proprietary menthol rubs. If you cannot breathe through your nose, breathe through your mouth and humidify the room. Never on any account sniff salt water, nor put any chemicals in your nose unless prescribed by a doctor: they can cause long-term damage and recurrent nasal blockage.

**Apnoea**  The name for this condition is derived from the ancient Greek word meaning breathlessness. It is a rare but troublesome complaint that causes severe long-term broken sleep, most often in overweight men. When the sufferer falls asleep, an obstruction in the air passages of the throat prevents him breathing for ten or twenty seconds at a stretch. Then the controls for maintaining the body's chemistry force the sleeper to take two or three violent snorting breaths that almost wake him up. This whole performance is repeated as a sequence for long periods of the night, so that the apnoea sufferer never really gets a sound night's rest, and in consequence is sleepy during the day.

The first line of treatment in most cases is to lose weight. However, in rare instances the obstruction to breathing during the night makes it difficult for blood to be pumped through the lungs, so that a strain is put on the heart. A surgical treatment has been devised whereby a special little tube can be inserted below the Adam's apple, to be used only at night. Sleep is then accompanied by a smooth succession of breaths, there is no sleepiness by day, and no strain on the heart.

Apnoea can also occur in children who have excessively large tonsils and adenoids. If it does, the child may be sleepy by day and

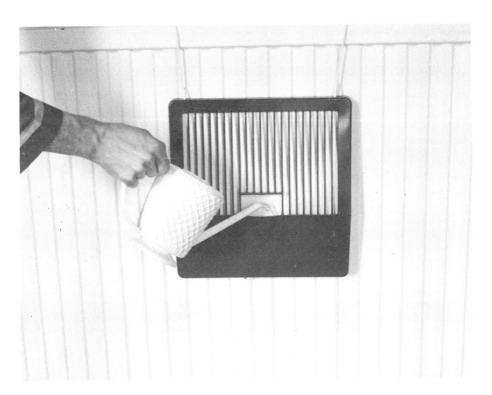

A persistent cough or wheezy chest can disturb sleep. Warm, humid aid – achieved here with a radiator and a humidifier – helps to soothe troubled breathing.

unable to concentrate on lessons at school. Breathing difficulties by day and by night will lead parents to decide that a visit to the family doctor is required. Although the operation for removal of tonsils and adenoids is less popular today than in former years, it may be recommended for your child so that he or she may breathe properly at night.

**Snoring** The very mention of snoring is guaranteed to provoke mirth. It should be noted that the snorts which punctuate periods of apnoea differ from ordinary snoring, in that the latter is usually in the form of a regular melody with only occasional variations.

It is the listener who complains, not the snorer. At least one person in ten is a snorer, both men and women of all ages. Snoring does no harm, though it may result in a dry mouth. The snorer, upon awakening, has difficulty in understanding how the alleged noise could have been so great if he himself slept through it. The sounds may have ranged from a gentle buzz or a low whistle to a prolonged roaring, reminiscent of a pneumatic drill. The marriage vows do not include a promise to endure snoring till death brings a parting and excessive snoring has been considered justification for divorce, at least in the United States. Snoring has also led to threats to kill the snorer by infuriated dwellers in the same tenement. Like aircraft noise, the seriousness of the effect upon the listener depends upon how readily the listener becomes annoyed.

The snorer should avoid evening alcohol and keep slim, but generally speaking, medical science has little to offer; and so it seems that friendly tolerance, ear-plugs or separate bedrooms must provide the answers. Innumerable devices have been patented as treatments. Snoring commonly occurs with your mouth open while lying on your back, so some of the devices have entailed elastic bandages for keeping the mouth closed. Another device was a small ball that emitted a squeaking noise when the snorer rolled on to his back, the noise being intended to prompt him to turn back on his side. One invention patented in the United States in 1961 involved a chin-strap with a battery-operated vibrator and an automatic alarm, both of which were designed to go off whenever the snorer's mouth opened during the night. Most of these must have been at least as disruptive of a partner's sleep as the snorer's own gentle sounds.

There are, of course, other common causes of insomnia, such as synthetic drugs, tobacco and alcohol, but these warrant the whole of the next chapter to themselves. Whatever the cause of your poor sleep, there is one question that is probably uppermost in your mind.

# How will insomnia affect me?

The most important advice we can offer you is that you need not worry that you will come to any serious harm on account of your poor sleep. If possible, you should come to accept that as you grow older you are not going to have the kind of sleep you did when you were young.

Your sleep probably is not as bad as you think, anyway. We really are all very inaccurate in our judgements as to how much we sleep. In Stanford in California, the sleep of 120 people who thought that they slept badly was compared by recording their electrical brain waves in the laboratory on some nights and by getting them to make their own estimates of how many hours they slept, or how many minutes it took them to fall asleep. While there were indeed a few who took a couple of hours to fall asleep, they were only the tiny minority. Most of the volunteers fell asleep within a matter of minutes, even though they felt that they usually took much longer. Likewise, although there were indeed some people who only slept about four hours in the night, those who *thought* that they generally slept only about four hours, but in fact slept considerably longer, were far more numerous.

Nevertheless, as we made clear in Chapter 2, there is more to sleep than just its duration. The laboratory sleep of those who believe they are poor sleepers does indeed contain more frequent awakenings through the night. Moreover, the body temperature of poor sleepers does not fall as low in the middle of the night as does the temperature of good sleepers, which is a sign that the poor sleepers are not getting so profound a degree of rest and are therefore unlikely to be getting such good conditions for a refreshing night's sleep.

We mentioned in Chapter 2 that the corticosteroid hormones, which hinder the renewal of the body's tissue during sleep, are

This graph illustrates the findings of the Californian study mentioned opposite. Comparison of the pairs of columns shows that most insomniacs in fact sleep longer than they think they do.

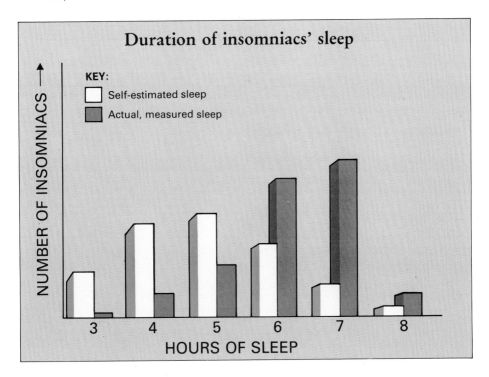

normally low during the night, begin to rise before sleep usually ends, and rise to high levels after breakfast. Some people, at least, who feel that their sleep is of poor quality have higher levels of corticosteroids all through the night, and by day too, than do those who feel that they have good quality sleep. So it is possible that poor sleep may provide less than ideal conditions for renewal of mind and body. This does not mean you will run down like a car battery that is being drained of energy without sufficient recharging. Your body and brain will restore themselves adequately whatever the quality of your sleep but may have more of a struggle to do so.

Your sleep may be bad just now or even always bad. Of itself, we must repeat, this will not harm you. If there is recent deterioration of your sleep for no obvious reason, accompanied by loss of energy and normal interest, then it is reasonable to see your doctor. Don't help yourself to sleeping pills that were prescribed years ago for someone else. Don't spend money on vitamin supplements or cranky devices like hop pillows and magnetic headbands, nor on clinics that claim to cure insomnia: it is much better to be advised first by your regular family doctor.

# 7. HOW DRUGS AFFECT YOUR SLEEP

We have stressed several times throughout the book that drugs can have a detrimental effect on your sleep: not only stimulant drugs, many of which are taken unwittingly every day; but also, ironically, sleeping drugs themselves; and, of course, the most heavily consumed sleep-inducing drug in the world, alcohol.

We will examine first the most obvious category of sleep-disturbers – the stimulants; then we will explain the ways in which different types of sleeping drugs work, and how they can have the opposite to their intended effect; and finally we will be offering guidelines for the safe and beneficial short-term use of sleeping pills.

## Drugs that keep you awake

### Nicotine

Nicotine is the commonest drug of addiction in the world, and most people are aware that its intake in the form of tobacco smoke is the cause of chest diseases, heart diseases, arterial diseases, digestive disorders and cancer. It is not so widely known that nicotine absorbed by inhalation of tobacco smoke also stimulates the nervous system, increases the depth of breathing and raises the blood pressure. It brings about the release of the hormone adrenaline (epinephrine) in the body, which, as we mentioned in Chapter 2, increases energy and liveliness and counteracts the effect of body-building hormones that restore us while we sleep.

After smoking a cigarette, the concentration of nicotine in the blood rises and, depending upon the individual, the next cigarette is not smoked until the level of nicotine has fallen considerably. If the amount of nicotine in cigarettes is deliberately halved, then the rate of smoking them just about doubles. Unknown to themselves, people smoke in a way that keeps the amount of nicotine in their tissues fairly constant. Desperate to get a last drag, and unaware that nicotine will disturb their sleep, many smoke at bedtime (a dangerous practice, in any case, that is a frequent cause of fires). Quite apart from the coughing and the wheezing from years of damage to the lungs from the tobacco, the nicotine acts on the brain cells to interfere with sleep and make it less deep or actually broken.

The nicotine in the body's tissues disappears only gradually during the first few hours of sleep, but just how rapidly varies a great deal. In someone whose urine is characteristically alkaline, the nicotine will persist in the body about four times as long as in someone whose urine is characteristically acid. (Whether the urine is acid or alkaline depends very much on the habitual diet.)

Whether you suffer from insomnia or not, we would strongly advise you to give up smoking.

## Caffeine

This is another widely consumed drug that keeps you awake. Coffee, of course, is a widely enjoyed drink that contains caffeine. If you want to enjoy a cup of coffee before bedtime without later being kept awake, decaffeinated coffees, that have very little, if any, stimu-

Most people are aware that caffeine in coffee is a stimulant drug. It is not so widely known that the nicotine inhaled from tobacco smoke can also disturb sleep.

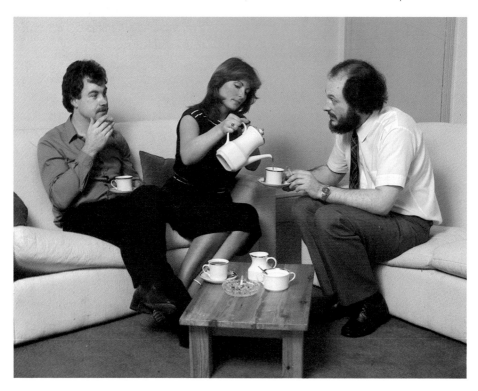

lating effect, are readily available.

Many people do not realize that tea, especially strong tea, also contains a lot of caffeine, together with a related chemical called theophylline. They are both drugs that increase feelings of energy, increase the body's temperature and cause greater wakefulness. Even cocoa, often drunk at bedtime, contains quite a lot of caffeine.

Caffeine is also found in cola drinks, when it comes from the nuts of *Cola acuminata* (guru nuts) that give the drink its distinctive flavour. We once had a patient, a middle-aged man, who came and spent some weeks in Edinburgh so that we could help him sleep better. He was from West Africa and, in that hot climate, he had for a long time made it a habit to quaff about seven bottles of cola drink each evening. The practice was not the only reason why he was a bad sleeper, but certainly contributed towards it.

Many over-the-counter preparations, especially pain-killers, contain caffeine, so it is always worth checking their contents before taking them in the evening or at night.

### Prescribed drugs

A few drugs deliberately prescribed can act as disturbers of sleep. Several antidepressant drugs make people have sudden jumps of the body at night, while a few, such as viloxazine (Vivalan) actually increase wakefulness in a manner similar to caffeine.

Slimming pills also keep you awake; the most widely used having been drugs like dexamphetamine (Dexedrine) or phenmetrazine (Preludin). They are very powerful drugs for disturbing sleep and keeping you awake, as well as for taking away your appetite for the first couple of weeks of intake. Apart from ruining your sleep, slimming by means of pills is not a good idea anyway, since as soon as you stop taking them you will probably put back on all the weight you have lost. It is far better to lose weight by putting yourself on a calorie-controlled diet. But before going to all this trouble, perhaps just to lose the odd pound so you can fit into the latest fashionable clothes, it would be worth while to read the next chapter, which reveals some interesting links between food, your weight and your sleep.

The commonest prescribed drugs associated with disturbance of sleep are the diuretic or water-losing drugs. There are many different diuretic drugs, but they are all designed to remove excess fluid from the body, and are often used in the treatment of heart trouble or high blood pressure. Inevitably they mean getting up to pass water more often at night. A urine bottle or chamber pot kept beside the bed will minimize the disturbance to your sleep.

### Increased sensitivity with age
It is important to realize that, just as natural ageing is associated with spontaneously more broken sleep, so the older brain becomes more sensitive to drugs that affect sleep or wakefulness. Many young people drink coffee or smoke cigarettes in the evening, or even at bedtime with no adverse effect on their sleep. Young people in their twenties usually sleep so well that nothing will disturb them. Should they continue their habits of drinking coffee and smoking into their thirties, they may wonder why they begin to have difficulty in falling asleep and why their sleep at night is restless. The explanation lies in the fact that their sleep is now being disturbed by the caffeine in their coffee, or by the nicotine in their cigarettes, because their brains have now become more sensitive to these stimulant drugs than when they were younger.

The older you are, the more sensitive you will be to sleeping drugs also. And it is to these that we shall now turn our attention.

# Drugs that send you to sleep

As far back as recorded history goes, men and women have sought sleep – and release into hallucinatory states – by means of naturally occuring drugs. The Aztecs of Central America used sacred mushrooms; and from the East came hashish, derived from the plant *Cannabis sativa*, and opium, from the poppy. But among all the old sleep-inducing potions, those made from the root of the mandrake plant enjoyed the greatest popularity. The mandrake, a member of the potato family, is often shaped as if it had arms and legs, and this characteristic has made it the subject of many legends. The mandrake contains hyoscine, a drug related to belladonna, which in large doses is dangerous.

The use of these naturally occuring drugs to promote sleep has now been superceded in developed countries by synthetic chemical drugs. All the chemical sleeping drugs described in this chapter are prescription drugs. Over-the-counter, off-prescription preparations are nearly all ineffective. We should point out here that a prescribed drug should be taken only by the person for whom it was prescribed, never in quantities larger than prescribed, and always kept out of reach of children.

Prescribed drugs generally have two names: the approved name of the chemical, and the trade name. We will be referring to all drugs by their approved name, and to some, where appropriate, also by their trade name, which is always written with a capital first letter. Many trade names differ from country to country, so to avoid complicating the text we have included an appendix on page 116 that lists the approved and trade names in several countries of all the drugs mentioned in the book.

## The first chemical sleeping drugs

By the nineteenth century the rise of modern chemistry began to bring artificial chemical agents which, though less romantic than those of the Middle Ages, were safer and more effective.

**Bromides**   In England in 1857 Sir Charles Locock introduced bromides into medicine for the treatment of epilepsy, and they were found to cause drowsiness. The use of bromides continued well into the twentieth century but today they have rightly nearly disappeared. Though effective in reducing epileptic seizures, the bromides were not really suitable for use as sleeping drugs, or hypnotics, as they are sometimes called, since only by gradual accumulation over a period of days and weeks can they cause drowsiness, and the effect is present by day as well as by night, affecting both alertness and general health.

**Paraldehyde**   This is a colourless liquid that smells strongly and has a burning taste. It used to be given with various masking agents to camouflage the taste and smell and up until a few years ago it still figured in the official list of drugs available in Britain as the sleeping draught, *Haustus Paraldehydi*. Some patients grew to love the way it burned their throat like whisky.

Paraldehyde could also be injected through a syringe, a practice that has continued with diminishing frequency up to the present day. It is an effective drug for inducing sleep and for relieving the insomnia caused by the withdrawal of alcohol. But the great disadvantage of paraldehyde is that some of it leaves the body again as vapour through the lungs so that the whole house, or a whole hospital, reeks of paraldehyde if anyone present has received it in the last twelve hours.

**Chloral hydrate**   This chemical compound came into use as a sleeping drug in the nineteenth century, and in a modified form it is still used today in proprietary pills such as Welldorm, Noctec and Triclofos. It was first prepared by the chemist, Baron Justus von Leibig, in Munich in 1832. Whereas other sleeping drugs, such as the bromides, had a great many other unwanted side-effects, chloral had a more selective action, and in this respect was the forerunner of modern sleeping drugs. It was synthesized by Leibig from chloroform and an alkali, and was wrongly thought to release chloroform (then recently introduced for use in anaesthesia) into the bloodstream. It was chloral hydrate, mixed into alcoholic drinks, that furnished the original Mickey Finn knock-out draught. The nineteenth-century Pre-Raphaelite painter and poet, Dante Gabriel Rossetti, was thought to have been a chloral addict.

Chloral, however, remains an effective and safe hypnotic, of which there is little criticism; though because it is old, little money has been invested to carry out the kind of careful research that is devoted to modern sleeping drugs, and so there is perhaps some deficiency of critical research into the merits of chloral.

The $1/2$–1 g dosage for adults is very large compared with the minute quantities of modern sleeping drugs, which seem to have a way of latching on to the nerve cells so that incredibly small quantities can have widespread effects.

## The barbiturates

The most famous sleeping pills in the twentieth century have been the barbiturates. In Berlin in 1864, Adolf von Baeyer created barbituric acid in his chemical laboratory, making it from malonic acid and urea. He went out to celebrate his achievement at a local drinking house much favoured by artillery officers and did so on the Day of St Barbara – the patron saint of artillery officers – and so from the words 'Barbara' and 'urea' was born the word 'barbiturate'.

Then in 1903, Fischer and von Mering, again working in Berlin, made barbitone, the old Veronal. Barbitone was the first barbiturate sleeping drug, and its use spread rapidly across the world. Sure enough, it made people sleep; but once taken into the body, it was many days before it left again, and so people were sleepy all day as well as at night.

In 1912 came phenobarbitone (Luminal), perhaps the most famous of them all, which was very widely prescribed not only to induce sleep and soothe the nerves of insomniacs by day, but much more effectively to treat epilepsy. Like barbitone, phenobarbitone was not really a suitable drug for making people sleep at night, because there was almost as much left in the body at breakfast-time as there had been before midnight.

There then followed a number of shorter-acting barbiturates, that are still prescribed today, and are known by trade names such as Sodium Amytal, Nembutal, and Soneryl. These later barbiturates were very effective in relieving anxiety and inducing sleep.

Variations were introduced in which the anxiety-relieving effects of a barbiturate were supposed to be preserved while the sleep-inducing effects were counteracted by the addition of dexamphetamine, a drug causing wakefulness. These mixtures, of which the so-called 'purple hearts' were the best known, soon became recognized as drugs that would give a 'high', and addiction and trafficking developed. Considerable quantities of barbiturates are still dispensed throughout the world, mainly to elderly people who have been reluctant to give up the crutch they have known for so many years. Unfortunately the barbiturates are dangerous in overdose, and the rate of deaths per prescription from barbiturates has risen in recent years, despite an overall reduction in their prescribing. And, as we will be explaining later on in the chapter, continuing use of barbiturates leads to physical dependence on the drug.

## The non-barbiturates

As it became recognized that barbiturates were liable to abuse and dependence, with unpleasant symptoms when they were stopped after regular intake, a variety of newer compounds was introduced, such as glutethimide (Doriden), meprobamate (Equanil) and the ill-fated thalidomide. Another was methaqualone: the mandrakes of olden times were to be succeeded by the new Mandrax, a pill containing methaqualone mixed with a drug called diphenhydramine. Introduced in the 1960s, Mandrax was an instant success, and most especially among drug abusers who found in it another avenue to a quick 'high'. Both Mandrax and barbiturates became popular targets for drug pushers, who would often break into pharmacists' shops in order to steal these drugs and then sell them; and so Mandrax, after a few dizzy years of success, has departed from the prescribing scene – even more rapidly than the barbiturates.

There have been recent claims made by one or two researchers in the United States that pills containing the amino acid tryptophan, found naturally in food protein, are effective in promoting sleep. Our research in Edinburgh, however, does not confirm these claims. We will be discussing the effects of tryptophan in detail in the next chapter.

## The benzodiazepines

In 1957 a new drug was discovered called chlordiazepoxide, that a few years later came to be sold as Librium. A great many chemically related drugs have followed, belonging to the general class known as benzodiazepines. They all have the same actions in human beings, of relieving anxiety and promoting sleep. However, they differ in three respects: in the dosage necessary; in the further chemical compounds into which they are changed once they have entered the body; and in the persistence in the body both of the original compound and of the changed compounds. Some, like diazepam (Valium) and flurazepam (Dalmane) are like the barbiturate phenobarbitone in that, with repeated intake, the concentrations of drug in the tissues build up cumulatively until eventually a plateau is reached. This means that almost as much drug is affecting the brain by day as by night. Others, especially some of the newer ones like lormetazepam (Noctamid), when taken at bedtime, do not accumulate in the same way, about half of a bedtime dose being gone by breakfast-time.

The benzodiazepines are very much safer drugs than their predecessors. An overdose of most barbiturates can lead to death, whereas an overdose of benzodiazepine drugs virtually never does. One of the curious features of benzodiazepines is that if somebody takes twenty pills of, say, nitrazepam (Mogadon) then the next morning they do not appear very much more doped than if they had taken only two or three (though they will stay dopey for longer). The explanation seems to be that the molecules of the drug can only act on the brain cells by attaching themselves to certain positions, called 'receptors'. The number of these receptors is very limited, so that if they are occupied nearly to the full by a small intake of the drug, there is not much scope for further action even if a very large quantity has been taken. This would also explain why amazingly small doses of some of the benzodiazepines are effective. Whereas the dose of chloral hydrate might be 1 g, and the dose of a barbiturate such as amylobarbitone sodium (Sodium Amytal) 200 mg, the dose of one of the newer and modified benzodiazepines called triazolam (Halcion) is 0.125 mg.

It is the safety factor that is the greatest merit in the benzodiazepines. They are not knock-out drops in the way that the barbiturates or Mandrax were, and they do not give a 'high', and so have held little attraction for drug abusers and pushers. It would be wrong, however, to imagine that there are not some people who abuse benzodiazepines, or to think that dependence does not develop.

Dependence on these drugs is common, but the severity both of the dependence and of the symptoms on the withdrawal of benzodiazepines is much milder than after prolonged intake of a barbiturate. This is partly because most of the benzodiazepines, like flurazepam (Dalmane) or nitrazepam (Mogadon), are slowly eliminated from the body's tissues, so that the let-down is gradual.

The newer benzodiazepines, like lormetazepam (Noctamid), leave the body faster but give a sharper let-down on withdrawal. Taken regularly, benzodiazepines do lead to dependence, but the social effects are few compared with dependence upon alcohol, and the dangers smaller than with barbiturates.

Benzodiazepines have been very successful in financial terms, but many of us in the medical profession believe that they have been greatly overprescribed. Even though for commercial purposes some are advertized as sleeping pills and some as tranquillizers to soothe the nerves by day, all benzodiazepines have both these effects.

### Alcohol

People don't usually think of alcohol as a drug, but of course that's exactly what it is. Alcohol certainly makes many of us sleepy, at least if we take it in the evening; and there are those who like to take a hot toddy or some other small but strong drink at bedtime, with a view to promoting sleep. In spite of its effectiveness in bringing on sleep, alcohol is not only a cause of great social problems, but is also a leading cause of *bad* sleep. It gets you to sleep more quickly, but you pay for it later through the rebound that will be described in the next section, as well as through gastritis, lack of appetite in the morning, and often a headache as well.

# The unwanted effects of some sleeping drugs

The most familiar among all the sleep-inducers is alcohol, and everyone knows that a large quantity of alcohol can make you fall over while walking, or have an accident while driving a car. Common sense and a lot of research tell us that smaller quantities of alcohol have the same kinds of effect but in smaller degree, and that the effects are proportional to how much drink has been consumed. If you drink only a really small amount – say $^1/_2$ pint/275 ml of beer – then by an extra effort of concentration you can compensate in part for the effects of the alcohol, but only to a limited extent.

All the other sleeping drugs resemble alcohol. They promote sleep as well as altering its detailed composition; usually, for example, by reducing the proportion of time you normally spend in paradoxical sleep (not that you will be in any way aware of this, nor be harmed in any way as a result). In addition, they reduce anxiety; they make us unsteady on our feet, slurred in our speech, inclined to have accidents; and they impair our usual good judgement.

## Impaired judgement

One way of finding out if someone's abilities are impaired by alcohol is to go out in a car driven by that person. We might not all want to. Another way is to ask someone who has been drinking to walk carefully, heel to toe, along a line. Tests of skilful co-ordination like this are also used to see whether sleeping pills taken at bedtime leave unwanted effects during the next day. We have conducted many such experiments at our Edinburgh laboratories.

On the nights before the daytime tests our volunteers take a pill before going to bed. All the pills look identical, but, known only to us, some are inactive and others are sleeping pills of varying types. The volunteers come for two hours of tests in the morning, two hours of tests in the middle of the day and two hours of tests in the late afternoon.

We ask them to pick up lead shot pellets as fast as they can and fit them into an awkward vertical tube at high speed for two minutes, to see how many they can cram in. We ask them to deal playing cards into two boxes as fast as they can. We ask them to sit with headphones on for an hour while performing a very boring task, during which they are supposed to listen for occasional special noises played through the headphones, and then to press a button when the noises are heard. This test is designed to see how well they can maintain concentration despite the boredom. Tests like these can tell us when someone has taken a sleeping pill the night before.

Many of the modern benzodiazepine sleeping drugs, such as triazolam (Halcion) or lormetazepam (Noctamid), have largely disappeared from the body's tissues by breakfast-time and there may be little or no impairment of skill the next day, or, at the most, only first thing in the morning. Other sleeping drugs, like flurazepam (Dalmane) – also a benzodiazepine, if taken regularly, can build up in the tissues and cause sustained impairment of abilities throughout the day. This is not yet fully realized by all doctors and flurazepam remains very widely prescribed, especially in the United States.

Many people take alcohol, barbiturates or benzodiazepines to calm themselves during the day. We all know how anxiety can make us

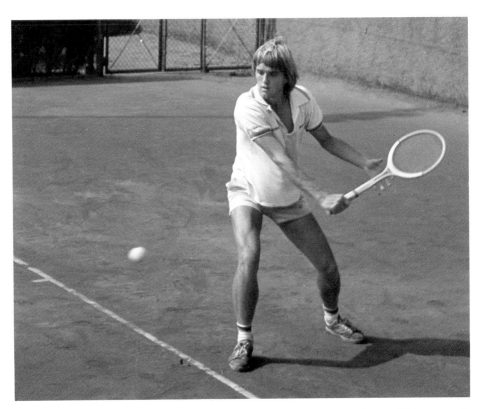

Both sleeping pills and alcohol impair judgement. Someone who takes a drink to steady the nerves will not perform as well as he would have done had he abstained.

inefficient. It is the basis of the old saying about the more haste the less speed. The tennis player who can watch the ball to the middle of his racquet when he is relaxed, may play badly in front of a crowd on a great occasion, due to nerves. Some argue therefore that if this anxious tennis player were to have a pre-match measure of whisky, or take a small dose of a barbiturate or a benzodiazepine – all of which diminish anxiety – then he would play better than he otherwise might. It makes a plausible story: taking a drink to steady the nerves.

Unfortunately the facts of real life do not support this rationale for taking alcohol, barbiturates or benzodiazepines. In general, bad nerves plus drugs are worse than bad nerves alone, as far as objective skill is concerned, even if subjective experiences are altered in a more pleasurable way. In other words, the tennis player who takes something for his nerves will actually play worse than if he had abstained, although the drug may cause him to think he has played better.

Just as the original Mickey Finn mixture of alcohol and chloral was a veritable bombshell, so alcoholic drinks taken on top of modern sleeping pills, such as the benzodiazepines, can cause a greater degree of incapacity than would be caused just by the sum of their parts.

**Irritability and aggression**
If you take a drink in the peaceful surroundings of your evening armchair, you may fall asleep. Alcohol consumed in the afternoon by spectators at the sports stadium, for example, does not always lead to sleepiness; it can lead to aggressive behaviour and fighting. Everything depends on the circumstances. And just as people may say foolish and hurtful things, and get into fights after drinking alcohol, so they may after taking the other drugs that promote sleepiness. The drugs may be sold to soothe the nerves, but – as we have seen – they also blunt your judgement; and on occasions can lead to unpredictable outbursts of temper under provocation. Careful laboratory tests have shown that when deliberately provoked in conversation, people's tempers are more easily unleashed when they have taken a pill containing chlordiazepoxide (Librium) than when they have taken an identical-looking pill that is inactive, even though they do not know what the pills contain.

In our own research we conducted a large study with twenty-one volunteers over about nine months, during which they took, for stretches of weeks at a time, one kind of pill or another. We coded the pills so that neither we nor the volunteers knew which drug they were taking at the time they were taking it.

During the 450 volunteer-weeks of the study there were seven serious incidents. There was the woman who started weeping and quarrelling with the employer she had worked with quite happily for years. There was the housewife who became more and more depressed and irritable and filled with impulses to murder a member of her family. Another housewife got into other difficulties by becoming bad tempered at home.

When eventually we broke the code and learned who had been taking which drugs when, we discovered that all the seven incidents had occurred when the volunteers involved had been taking 30 mg flurazepam (Dalmane) at bedtime. The Dalmane-taking had only occupied 63 out of the 450 weeks. During the other weeks either inactive pills or a more modern sleeping pill – lormetazepam (Noctamid) – had been taken as the alternative. It could not be explained by chance and we had to conclude that the Dalmane had actually been the cause of the trouble. The reason why this particular drug is best avoided is because it accumulates in the body's tissues as the days go by, and so there is bound to be a large quantity active throughout the day, instead of just at night.

## Withdrawal rebounds

Most of you will have heard of the DTs, or *delirium tremens*. What typically happens is that a heavy drinker of alcohol falls ill and so is prevented from having his usual drink. Then a couple of nights later he becomes restless, twitching, unable to sleep, all of a tremble, filled with terror at the sight of horrible visions, and possibly even has epileptic seizures. Just the same can happen when accustomed heavy intake of barbiturates stops, or any other sleeping pill, though the picture is less severe after taking the benzodiazepines. DTs is the extreme result, but the same troubles arise to a lesser degree whenever any sleeping drug is stopped after being taken regularly in the pre-scribed dosage.

Why should this happen? It is because the brain is always adapting, changing to meet new circumstances, so that if it finds itself in the presence of a strange chemical never intended by Nature to be present in the brain fluids, it adapts itself to counteract the effects of the chemical.

We all have a certain natural degree of anxiety. We all have an individual natural restlessness as part of our constitution. If a drug that reduces anxiety and restlessness is taken for weeks, then the brain gradually changes its own internal machinery over the same period, as if to try and bring back the natural level of anxiety and restlessness. That means there is, as it were, new equipment in the brain for making us more anxious, more restless. If the drug is now stopped, we are lumbered with the new equipment, and, without the soothing drug, are now more anxious and more restless than we would have been had we never taken the drug.

The adaptational change that brings about the new equipment in the brain to counteract the effect of the drug, is called 'tolerance'. Tolerance means that whereas when we first took a sleeping pill it really knocked us out, by the time we have got used to taking it regularly, it has lost much of its old intensity of effect. Any sleeping pill to some extent 'loses its effect' as a result of tolerance, and so when the drug is no longer taken, the new counteracting equipment in the brain causes a rebound into the opposite of the drug's effect.

A drug that makes you fall asleep more quickly, and have longer sleep, makes you have less paradoxical sleep and less anxiety, will, when you stop taking it, make you experience prolonged delay in getting to sleep, have shortened hours of sleep, lots of paradoxical sleep, and lots of anxiety, with vivid dreams and nightmares. These effects will be most severe in the first few nights following the stopping of some drugs, a bit more delayed after others; but it is certain that they will be unpleasant and will persist in diminishing degree for a couple of months. So, stopping sleeping drugs can be difficult!

Just how sharp and immediate this rebound is varies according to the drug. Stopping flurazepam (Dalmane), for example, does not lead to such severe rebound effects as stopping many other sleeping drugs, because flurazepam accumulates in the tissues over a period of many days and correspondingly takes a period of many days to leave the tissues, so allowing a gradual let-down.

Alcohol gives a sharp rebound, because it is rapidly destroyed in the body over a period of a few hours. You have probably had the experience of drinking more than usual in the evening and then getting something of a rebound, or withdrawal reaction, causing you

This shows the withdrawal rebound after weeks of taking one of the short-acting sleeping drugs. The rebound effects after prolonged intake include difficulty in getting to sleep, fewer hours of sleep and more nightmares.

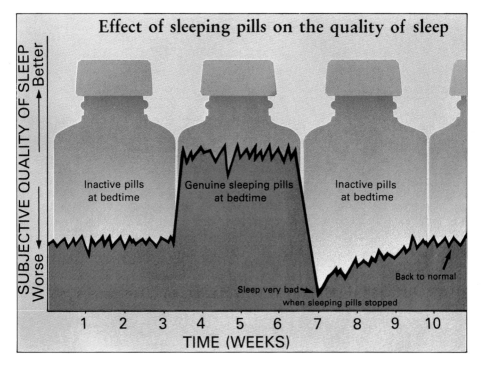

Effect of sleeping pills on the quality of sleep

SUBJECTIVE QUALITY OF SLEEP
Better
Worse

Inactive pills at bedtime

Genuine sleeping pills at bedtime

Inactive pills at bedtime

Sleep very bad when sleeping pills stopped

Back to normal

TIME (WEEKS)
1 2 3 4 5 6 7 8 9 10

to wake in the small hours of the morning. The real alcoholic may wake up not just earlier than usual, but positively trembling. You also know that someone who drinks a whole bottle of gin regularly each evening is taking a large dose of a potent drug. The drug is one that induces sleep and relieves anxiety. If someone does this week after week then, before long, he is trembling each morning and dying to have another drink. If somehow he were forced to abstain until the evening he would be extremely anxious throughout the day until at last he got his evening drink.

In recent years we have realized the disadvantages of cumulative drugs like flurazepam; and one of the newer drugs, triazolam (Halcion) was introduced partly because, if taken at bedtime to induce sleep, it would virtually be gone from the body by morning. It is destroyed in the body just about as rapidly as alcohol. In many ways it is a sensible choice, but in our research in Edinburgh we have found that if, for three weeks, volunteers take a large dose of triazolam nightly at bedtime, then the effect on them by day is very similar to the effect of alcohol as far as anxiety is concerned (although triazolam is very much safer for the liver and the body's tissues). When people take a large dose of triazolam each evening for three weeks they become more and more anxious by day and this must be attributed to a rebound effect in the daytime as a result of repeated intake of the drug at bedtime. We must emphasize that we were using a larger-than-usual dose of 0.5 mg of triazolam and that if only 0.125 mg were used, we would not expect trouble to arise.

However, our experience with triazolam, as a very short-acting sleeping drug, and our unfortunate experiences with flurazepam as a very long-acting sleeping pill, lead us to favour one of the medium short-acting drugs as probably providing the best compromise for general use. A drug like lormetazepam (Noctamid), 1 mg, taken at bedtime is half gone from the body by breakfast time and, at the moment, seems to us to be the most sensible available. This does not mean, though, that after several weeks of regular intake, there will not be the inevitable nights of bad sleep in the first couple of weeks after stopping the drug.

# The right sleeping drugs for short-term use

So, to sum up, there is a choice between two different types of sleeping drug. On the one hand are the older benzodiazepines, such as diazepam (Valium) and flurazepam (Dalmane) and barbiturates, such as phenobarbitone (Luminal), all of which will promote sleep and impair your efficiency round the clock, and, when stopped, not be followed by a sharp rebound. While on the other hand are the modern short-acting benzodiazepines such as lormetazepam (Noctamid), that leave you bright and alert by day, but which give you quite a sharp shock as soon as you try to stop taking them after a period of continued use. Of the two types we think the latter is preferable.

The fact that prior consumption of sleeping drugs can make sleep even worse than it would have been provides an obvious argument against taking them. However, as this effect is very dependent on the number of consecutive nights you take the drug, there are times when short-term use can be beneficial. Temporary crises such as the death of a close relative or friend, or an operation, can deprive you of the comfort of sleep when you need it. Taking a sleeping pill for a couple of nights may prevent this and enable you to cope with the worst period of the crisis, without having to suffer any noticeable withdrawal rebound. But remember that the more nights you take sleeping pills, the greater the rebound when you stop. As a general rule, we would advise you to try not to take them for more than two or three nights successively. But whether to take them for a few days until a crisis has passed, or for longer, depends on your own special circumstances and is ultimately a matter for you and your family doctor to decide upon.

If you have been taking sleeping drugs for a week or several weeks, or even longer, then you must expect to sleep badly in the weeks after stopping the drug. Your sleep will eventually return to its natural pattern but it may take six to eight weeks, and they can be difficult weeks. Being forewarned is being prepared. Tenacity may be required, but a successful return to natural sleep is well worth the effort.

Drugs are not the only substances we consume that affect the way we sleep. Food and drink also play a part, as does, indeed, our weight; exactly how and to what extent, we shall attempt to show in the next chapter.

# 8. FATNESS, FOOD AND SLEEP

## Your weight affects how long you sleep

We mentioned in Chapter 6 that being of a nervous disposition is associated with poorer sleep, at least as people judge their sleep for themselves. Being worried not only interferes with sleep, for most of us it also takes away the appetite for food (though there are people who find comfort in eating and who tend to overeat when anxious). The psychiatrist who has most notably called attention to the relationship between people's weight and how much they sleep is Prof Arthur Crisp of London. In January 1976, he, together with a colleague, published in the *British Medical Journal* an article describing their investigation into the relationship between, on the one hand, how people felt about their own emotions, and their height and weight, on the other. The article was called 'Jolly Fat', because it showed that people who were fatter were also people who were happier.

Prof Crisp and his team picked out from the list of a family doctors' practice in south London the names of a thousand men and women, simply on the basis of where their names fell in the alphabet. They had to be aged between forty and sixty-five. The 70 per cent who were prepared to co-operate attended the doctors' surgery and had their heights and body weights carefully measured. They then completed what is called the Middlesex Hospital Questionnaire, which was designed to measure how anxious each person normally felt himself or herself to be, how depressed they felt they generally were, and so on. Making allowance for height, people were classified into those who were overweight by 20 per cent, those who were overweight by 40 per cent or more, and those who were not overweight.

The questionnaire revealed that on average the fat people were happier people in their own eyes than those of leaner build. Since, as we have seen, being happy is associated with good sleep, and being anxious and depressed is associated with poor sleep, fat people can be expected to sleep better than thin people.

A few years ago at Edinburgh we were conducting research into the normal, undrugged sleep of middle-aged people of stable body weight, and used the EEG (see Chapter 3) to record their sleep throughout twenty nights each. Making allowance for their height and whether they were of large, medium or small body frame, we used the Metropolitan Life Assurance weight tables (see page 94) to assess each volunteer's ideal body weight. The more they were above their ideal weight, the longer they slept at nights in the laboratory, and if they were underweight, they slept less than other average people.

Their weight seemed also to have governed the running of their biological clocks. You will remember the 100-minute ultradian rhythm during sleep; we were interested to find that the volunteers who were above ideal body weight had cycles that were longer than the usual 100 minutes, and those who were below had shorter cycles.

So we found, as Crisp's work had suggested, that fat people do indeed sleep longer. We had judged how fat our volunteers were by relating their weight to their height. Just taking their gross body weight into account, without considering height, we found that the heavier people spent proportionately more of the night in paradoxical sleep.

In this kind of sleep, the muscles are profoundly relaxed, that is to say they are getting their most extreme rest. The heavier you are, the more energy you have to expend every day, partly for lifting your body up hills and out of chairs, but more especially just for sustaining posture, holding your head upright and back straight. So it may be that heavy people take more paradoxical sleep at night to give their muscles extra rest after the heavier work by day – though this is just an educated guess.

## You lose sleep when you lose weight

Prof Crisp and his colleague, Dr Stonehill, used to run a slimming clinic for severely overweight people, and they asked their patients to keep a regular note of how much they slept. They found that as the fat people got thinner, they thought they slept less. Crisp and his colleagues found the clearest example of this in patients who manifest anorexia nervosa, a condition of voluntary starvation. The sleep of these patients was measured using the EEG all night at a time when they were being fed a good diet. First of all, sleep was measured while they were very thin and then, weeks later, on the same diet, sleep was measured again when they had reached normal weight. The more weight they put on, the more they slept. When they had been very thin they had tended to wake early and lie awake for long periods before getting up. When returned to their normal weight they slept soundly through the later hours of the night.

Crisp and Stonehill asked another question: when people attend a psychiatric clinic and describe how they have been sleeping less well lately, to what extent might this be a consequence simply of weight loss? To find the answer they arranged their own psychiatric clinic in the following way. Every new outpatient was seen by someone who found out whether body weight had recently been steady, whether there had been a loss of weight, or whether there had been a gain. Quite independently, someone else decided after questioning the patient whether there had been some recent change in sleep, such as waking more in the night and sleeping less, or sleeping more than usual. Finally the psychiatrist saw the patient and at the end of the interview made a judgement of the patient's mood in terms of general happiness or unhappiness. When all three sets of data were subsequently put together, it emerged that people who had recently lost weight were the same people who described sleeping less in recent times and especially waking up earlier than usual; and all this proved to be unrelated to their mood of happiness or unhappiness. Crisp and Stonehill concluded that the poor sleep which frequently accompanies spells of depression can largely be attributed not to the depression itself, with its unhappy thoughts, but to sheer loss of body weight.

## What is the best weight for you?
In summary, therefore, people who are rather overweight tend to consider themselves to be happier people, and to sleep more than those who are underweight. Getting very thin is bad for your body anyway, but it is particularly bad for sleep.

We are not advocating that you get fat. Extremes in matters of health are generally best avoided. Apart from significantly increasing the risk of developing heart trouble and arthritis, severe obesity may also be detrimental to sleep. The sheer weight of fat in the abdomen can restrict night-time breathing, and for reasons we do not yet fully understand, very overweight people can suffer from periodic breathlessness – or sleep apnoea (see page 70) – that constantly disrupts their sleep throughout the night.

However, if you are under your ideal weight according to the weight table overleaf and you feel your sleep is not as good as you would like it to be, why not put on a pound or two? Or, if you are at your ideal weight or only 10 per cent or so above it, and you feel

## Weight table for men of 25 years and over (in indoor clothing)

| Height ft in (cm) | | Small frame lb | kg | Medium frame lb | kg | Large frame lb | kg |
|---|---|---|---|---|---|---|---|
| 5 1 | (155) | 112–120 | (51–54) | 118–129 | (54–59) | 126–141 | (57–64) |
| 5 2 | (157) | 115–123 | (52–56) | 121–133 | (55–60) | 129–144 | (59–65) |
| 5 3 | (160) | 118–126 | (54–57) | 124–136 | (56–62) | 132–148 | (60–67) |
| 5 4 | (163) | 121–129 | (55–58) | 127–139 | (58–63) | 135–152 | (61–69) |
| 5 5 | (165) | 124–133 | (56–60) | 130–143 | (59–65) | 138–156 | (63–71) |
| 5 6 | (168) | 128–137 | (58–62) | 134–147 | (61–67) | 142–161 | (64–73) |
| 5 7 | (170) | 132–141 | (60–64) | 138–152 | (63–69) | 147–166 | (67–75) |
| 5 8 | (173) | 136–145 | (62–66) | 142–156 | (64–71) | 151–170 | (68–77) |
| 5 9 | (175) | 140–150 | (63–68) | 146–160 | (66–73) | 155–174 | (70–79) |
| 5 10 | (178) | 144–154 | (65–70) | 150–165 | (68–75) | 159–179 | (72–81) |
| 5 11 | (180) | 148–158 | (67–72) | 154–170 | (70–77) | 164–184 | (74–83) |
| 6 0 | (183) | 152–162 | (69–74) | 158–175 | (72–80) | 168–189 | (76–86) |
| 6 1 | (185) | 156–167 | (71–76) | 162–180 | (74–82) | 173–194 | (78–88) |
| 6 2 | (188) | 160–171 | (73–78) | 167–185 | (76–84) | 178–199 | (81–90) |
| 6 3 | (190) | 164–175 | (74–80) | 172–190 | (78–86) | 182–204 | (83–92) |

## Weight table for women aged 25 and over (in indoor clothing)

(For women aged between 18 and 25 subtract 1 lb ($\frac{1}{2}$ kg) for each year under 25)

| Height ft in (cm) | | Small frame lb | kg | Medium frame lb | kg | Large frame lb | kg |
|---|---|---|---|---|---|---|---|
| 4 8 | (142) | 92–98 | (42–44) | 96–107 | (44–49) | 104–119 | (47–54) |
| 4 9 | (145) | 94–101 | (43–46) | 98–110 | (45–50) | 106–122 | (48–55) |
| 4 10 | (147) | 96–104 | (44–47) | 101–113 | (46–51) | 109–125 | (49–57) |
| 4 11 | (150) | 99–107 | (45–48) | 104–116 | (47–53) | 112–128 | (51–58) |
| 5 0 | (152) | 102–110 | (46–50) | 107–119 | (48–54) | 115–131 | (52–59) |
| 5 1 | (155) | 105–113 | (48–51) | 110–122 | (50–55) | 118–134 | (53–60) |
| 5 2 | (157) | 108–116 | (49–53) | 113–126 | (51–57) | 121–138 | (55–63) |
| 5 3 | (160) | 111–119 | (50–54) | 116–130 | (53–59) | 125–142 | (57–64) |
| 5 4 | (163) | 114–123 | (52–56) | 120–135 | (54–61) | 129–146 | (58–66) |
| 5 5 | (165) | 118–127 | (53–58) | 124–139 | (56–63) | 133–150 | (60–68) |
| 5 6 | (168) | 122–131 | (55–59) | 128–143 | (58–65) | 137–154 | (62–70) |
| 5 7 | (170) | 126–135 | (57–61) | 132–147 | (60–67) | 141–158 | (64–72) |
| 5 8 | (173) | 130–140 | (59–63) | 136–151 | (62–69) | 145–163 | (66–74) |
| 5 9 | (175) | 134–144 | (61–65) | 140–155 | (63–70) | 149–168 | (68–76) |
| 5 10 | (178) | 138–148 | (63–67) | 144–159 | (65–72) | 153–173 | (69–78) |

like slimming down – perhaps to make a good impression on the beach next summer – then think first whether a trim appearance is worth the risk of a period of shorter nights' sleep. To be a little on the chubby side can do you no harm, and may even help you to sleep better.

# How does food affect sleep?

### Lack of food
Going short of food leads to hunger pangs, the feelings of emptiness and discomfort from the stomach that are associated with actual contractions of the stomach wall as it seems to grope for food that is not there. These hunger pangs occur in bouts in the night, coming and going with the nocturnal 100-minute ultradian rhythm, and are accompanied by restless movements of the whole body. Human adults actually have plenty of food reserves stored away as fat, but babies do not have such reserves and it is more urgent that they steadily maintain their food intake. It does not need laboratory research workers to tell parents that their baby gets more and more restless and noisy if kept without food.

To see what would happen in adults we kept healthy young male volunteers without food for four days and nights at our laboratory (they were able to slake their thirst whenever they wanted), and sure enough they too slept less and less.

### Sleeping more after a meal
Being without food strengthens hunger pangs and disturbs sleep, and the converse is familiar to all of us who have felt sleepy after a large and satisfying meal. Any occasion for a feeling of general satisfaction, of achievement and gratification, is accompanied by relaxation and a sense of well-being, with a ready departure into somnolence. However, it is possible that the sleep of satiety is brought on by something more than just satisfaction of basic needs, for the hormones or enzymes that are released into the stomach and intestines to help with the digestion of food are in many cases the same chemicals as those that affect the working of the brain. The digestive enzyme known as cholecystokinin, for example, is nowadays believed to be one such chemical. When fat reaches the first part of the small intestine, called the duodenum, cholecystokinin is released to help with the digestion, and it has been claimed that when cholecystokinin is given to cats by injection, they fall asleep, just as they tend to do

after a meal. So it is possible that our digestive hormones pass via the bloodstream into the brain, to make us sleepy after a good meal.

## The tryptophan controversy
One of the constituents of protein in food is tryptophan, an amino acid, and you may have read in recent years the statements in newspapers, magazines, and books to the effect that tryptophan helps you fall asleep or makes you sleep more. We believe that some of these claims are based upon muddled thinking. There is indeed tryptophan in protein and $1/2$ lb/250 g of steak may make you sleepy after you've eaten it, but it can't be because of the tryptophan since the total amount in the steak is small and is only absorbed very slowly over a period of two, three or more hours while the steak is digested.

If you take pure tryptophan in the form of pills (Optimax, Pacitron or Trofan, for example), it is absorbed rapidly; but after it leaves the gut it has to go through the liver, where much of it gets destroyed, especially if there has been more tryptophan in the diet recently; and finally it has to go via the bloodstream into the brain. The amount that gets taken into the brain actually depends upon how much carbohydrate – which comes from starchy or sugary food – you have eaten at about the same time. The higher the carbohydrate content of the food, the more insulin hormone is passed into the bloodstream from the pancreas, and when there is a lot of insulin about, the tryptophan gets taken into the brain.

So just taking tryptophan pills, or eating a steak, gives no guarantee at all that significant quantities of the drug will reach your brain. Only if very large and unnatural quantities of tryptophan are taken by mouth accompanied by large amounts of carbohydrate can we be fairly certain that an excess is getting into the brain. When this is done people certainly do feel drowsy, their paradoxical sleep may come on earlier in the night than usual, and they can get rather more sleep than they would otherwise. However, the effect is a weak one, in no way comparable to taking a sleeping pill. We ourselves have been quite unable to confirm claims by researchers in Boston that smaller quantities of tryptophan, such as 1 g at bedtime (far more than there is in a steak) can make sleep come on a bit quicker.

OPPOSITE: Research has shown that an easily digested snack before bedtime can often lead to a more restful night's sleep. (See page 98.)

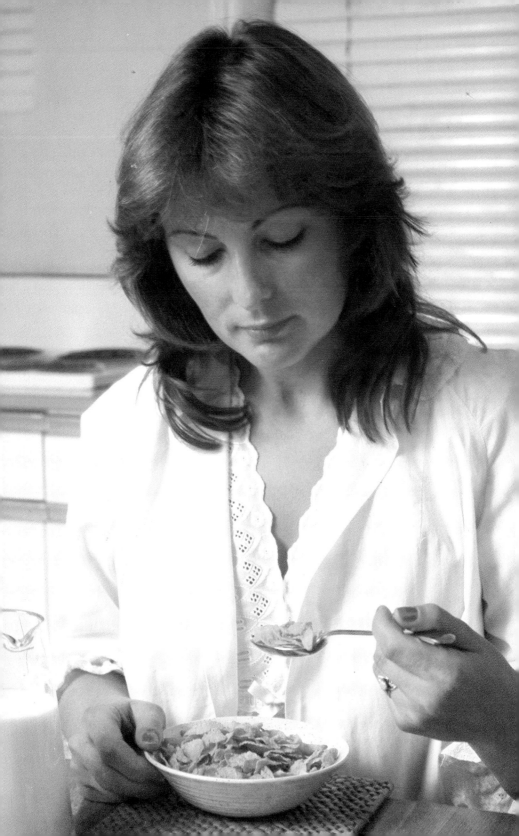

## Bedtime snacks and drinks

The debate over tryptophan is a relatively recent issue. For many years, though, it has been widely believed that a snack or hot milk drink at bedtime will be followed by a good night's sleep. Once again, the only way to find out if this is true is to test the theory in the sleep laboratory. The results have certainly been revealing.

In the 1930s, in the United States, Drs Laird and Drexel compared sleep after an easy-to-digest bedtime snack like cornflakes and milk, with a variety of hard-to-digest snacks, and found, not surprisingly perhaps, that hard-to-digest snacks were followed by restless sleep, whereas cornflakes and milk seemed to help sleep to be less restless, judging by the number of body movements during the night.

**Ovaltine**   In another immense study of sleep in Chicago, involving thousands of nights in which body movements were measured, the great American sleep researcher, Dr Nathanial Kleitman, compared the effects on sleep of a whole variety of bedtime snacks, ranging from plain water, bread and bread sandwiches containing cheese to plain milk, milk mixed with the malted bedtime food drink Ovaltine, and Ovaltine mixed with water. He found that there were fewest movements during the night among those who had drunk Ovaltine before going to bed, whether mixed with water or milk. Ovaltine is made from milk and cereal, so Kleitman's finding rather paralleled Laird and Drexel's results with cornflakes and milk.

**Horlicks**   This is another of the proprietary food drinks, for long famous as a proposed aid to sleep, which is again a malted milk drink prepared from cereal and milk products.

To test the effect of Horlicks on sleep, at Edinburgh we first tried two experiments, one with young and one with middle-aged volunteers. On some nights we gave them a yellow capsule that was actually inactive, though we told them that it contained a folk remedy for sleep, and on the other nights we gave them Horlicks mixed with hot milk. The young people slept so well on all their nights that nothing could have improved their sleep anyway, so no difference showed up with the Horlicks. The middle-aged people, however, slept quite a lot better after they had had Horlicks. There was a big difference in the amount of wakefulness in the later night particularly, the change being much more than could be accounted for by chance. The difference was striking, and more than we had originally expected; but there was a flaw in our method, as we were later to realize.

We then conducted a much bigger study in which sixteen volunteers had their EEGs recorded throughout the night, on a total of twenty nights each. On some nights they were just given the inactive 'folk remedy' capsule, on some nights milk, on some nights Horlicks mixed with milk, and on the other nights a flavoured drink specially concocted to contain no milk or cereal products, but the same calories and amounts of fat, carbohydrate and protein as Horlicks. Once again Horlicks emerged as best for sleep; but the difference, though greater than could be explained by chance, was a small one. It was also apparent that the rather unpalatable and specially made food drink seemed actually to disturb sleep. However, the most important factor to emerge lay in the customary habits of our volunteers.

When we had done the earlier study with the middle-aged people, we had asked for volunteers who would be willing to drink Horlicks at bedtime, so that, although we did not think of it at the time, we had probably been getting volunteers who were accustomed to having a bedtime drink or snack. So when they slept better during our test after drinking Horlicks this was due, as we later realized, to getting their usual nourishment at bedtime; and when they slept less well after an inactive capsule without any food value, they were relatively hungry and restless through the night because their stomachs were not used to being so empty while they slept.

In the second study we asked the volunteers to complete a diet questionnaire so that we could see the pattern of their normal evening eating habits at home. This confirmed that there was a link between how much was normally eaten in the later evening and the quality of sleep after a food drink in the laboratory. Those who normally ate little or nothing in the later evening at home slept best when they were given the inactive capsule with no food in it, and being unaccustomed to bedtime food supplements, their sleep was more disturbed after they had imbibed any of the food drinks before going to bed.

So where does all this research leave you if you want to know whether bedtime snacks and drinks will help or hinder your sleep? First of all, to go to bed feeling desperately hungry is not a good idea; but this is not to say that a full stomach will necessarily bring better sleep. It really depends on what you are used to: following your regular eating routine in the evening is the surest way to get the best sleep. In other words, don't have a large supper one evening and nothing on the next. If you are accustomed to eating in the evening, let it be something that is easily digested. Don't expect the best night's rest after a king-size hamburger and double portion of greasy French fries! Milk and the proprietary food drinks, being easily digestible sources of nourishment, probably are effective in helping you sleep, though their effect is not a strong one.

# 9. SOME SPECIAL SLEEP TROUBLES

Thus far we have dealt with the problems most people would immediately expect to find covered in a book called *Get a Better Night's Sleep* – namely, sleep loss, insomnia, nightmares, sleep-walking, and so on. There are, however, others that may not spring so readily to mind; unless, of course, either you, your partner or a member of your family are one of the many thousands who suffer from one or other of them. In this chapter we will be looking at the causes and the best way of coping with four special sleep troubles that we encounter frequently in the course of our work: bed-wetting; rhythmic movements, such as scratching and body-rocking; the night wanderings of the elderly; and sleeping too much. If you have trouble getting to sleep, this last condition no doubt sounds like a blessed state rather than something to worry about; but, as we shall be showing, it can prove to be quite a handicap.

## Bed-wetting (enuresis)

Most small infants wet their beds until they are three years old, many up to the age of five, and some when they are seven and older. Each child is different in its rate of development of night-time bladder control. Parents are human and it is not surprising that they may show their irritation on finding their five-year-old's bed wet yet again in the morning. But getting angry will only aggravate the situation by making the child feel guilty – unjustifiably – and thus possibly prolonging the bed-wetting. How it is that the sensations of a full bladder should wake us up in the night, we do not understand. We should try to appreciate how amazing it is that it should happen at all, rather than treat our children as a nuisance if they are a little slow in developing nocturnal bladder control. In any case, with time, the bed-wetting will cease, except in very unusual cases. Sometimes a child has been dry and starts wetting the bed again after an emotional crisis, such as the arrival of a new brother or sister, or a few days in hospital away from home. Again, parental patience and tolerance should be the order of the day.

A very few children have something wrong with their bladders or reflexes, so it is worth consulting a doctor if your child continues bed-wetting until school is started. Generally, though, there is no known cause, and occasionally bed-wetting may persist into the teens or early twenties before it finally stops of its own accord.

### Treatment

If tolerance, patience and understanding seem, in time, not to be helping the problem, then with your child's willing co-operation as an important factor, your doctor may suggest trying one of the following forms of treatment.

**Drugs**  Various drugs have been tried in the past in an attempt to prevent bed-wetting. It used to be thought that perhaps children who wet their bed were exceptionally deep sleepers and that if their sleep was kept light by drugs like dexamphetamine (Dexedrine), then the bed-wetting might cease. These drugs, however, are no longer in fashion.

Some of the drugs given to treat adults when they are ill with depression, like imipramine (Tofranil) and amitriptyline (Elavil or Tryptizol) have a number of side-effects, including interfering with the normal nervous reflexes that are required to begin urination. Older men can suddenly find themselves completely unable to pass urine when they have started on these drugs, and even women, for whom the act is usually simpler, may sometimes experience difficulty in getting going. This action of these antidepressant drugs has been applied to the treatment of bed-wetting, and it does seem that, on average, they do offer some benefits. However, the drugs are dangerous in overdose. The safest and most useful method of treatment is the so-called 'buzzer and pad' system.

**The 'buzzer and pad' system**  Wetting the bed really does occur during sleep. It is not that the child lies there awake, and just empties his bladder in order to be mischievous. Bed-wetting is one of those episodic disorders that occur most often in the early night, and almost always at the end of a period of deep slow-wave sleep.

Sleep is a time when learning does not readily occur; although the mental activity of sleep may be vivid, it is largely unremembered in the morning. The 'buzzer and pad' system, that can be prescribed by your family doctor, has to contend with this fact that it is difficult to learn while asleep.

The idea behind the treatment is that as soon as possible after the sheets become wet the child should awake. In order to achieve this a special pair of pads with metallic contacts, separated by a dry sheet, are placed beneath the sheet on which the child lies. A small difference of electrical potential is applied to the two pads, so that when the sheet between them becomes wet, an electric current can pass which triggers off a loud buzzer. Thus, when the bed is wet, the buzzer goes off, and the child wakes up.

In the language of the great Russian scientist, Pavlov, the loud noise is the unconditioned stimulus and the awakening is the unconditioned response. Shortly preceding the loud noise, however, there must have been internal signals from the distended bladder to the nervous system, which were unsuccessful in causing awakening. These signals, that always precede the unconditioned stimulus, fall into the category of what Pavlov called the conditioned stimulus. With repeated experience, over and over again, learning should take place (with luck), so that, when there is a strong conditioned stimulus of nervous messages from the tightly distended bladder, these alone should cause awakening, which could now be called a *conditioned* response. Hey presto! the full bladder in the night now causes awakening without the intervening wetting of the bed.

Complicated as this method sounds, it does work, though not quite always. The commonest reason for failure is probably the parents' lack of understanding of exactly what they have to do. If the child is woken up after wetting the bed he should get out and go to the lavatory to get rid of the urine that remains in his bladder, and a new, dry sheet should be placed between the pads. Another reason for failure is that the child simply sleeps through the noise of the buzzer, while all the rest of the household are awakened. A good technician can fix up an alternative device, by which a harmless electric shock can be delivered to the child's leg, in place of the buzzer.

Even so, there are a few young people, who, despite repeated experiences over many months of being woken up after the bed is wet, fail consistently to awaken before it is wet. For them, learning during sleep has not occurred. It is not their fault, it is just bad luck. There is another approach that can still be tried, and that is to find out when the bed-wetting characteristically occurs. It may, for example, nearly always take place about two hours after going to bed. If so, it can be arranged for the electric stimulus to wake up the sleeper after about an hour and three quarters, so that he can go and empty the bladder, and thereby avoid wetting the bed.

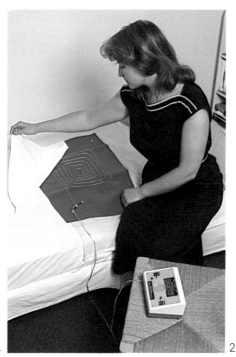
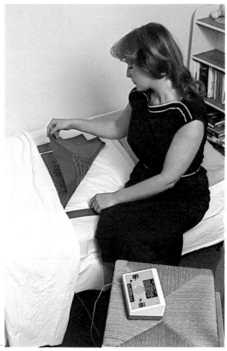

**The buzzer and pad system** 1. A small sheet is placed over the first pad to prevent the alarm going off until the bed is wet. 2. The second pad is laid on top, and the whole device finally covered by the sheet to be slept on.

Finally, it is worth repeating that no treatment for bed-wetting can work without the willing co-operation of your child.

# Rhythmic movements in the night

While we are asleep we lose many of our waking capabilities; but rhythmic movements are well within our compass and among these are scratching, tooth-grinding, and what is known as head-banging or body-rocking. In children and adults who are prone to make these rhythmic movements, they can occur at any time of night, though least often in deep slow-wave sleep.

### Scratching

We have studied the sleep of many people with itchy skin conditions such as eczema, and tried a number of drugs to relieve the itching, but without a great deal of success. Drugs that are specifically supposed to reduce itching seem to be no more effective than can be accounted for by the fact they make sleep rather heavier. Mostly, the scratching occurs when sleep is fairly light, and the scratching is certainly one of the reasons why some skin troubles are perpetuated and made worse, since scratched skin has to heal, and healing skin is often itchy. It is a vicious circle.

Keeping your nails short and scrupulously clean is obviously a sensible idea if you discover that you must have been scratching while asleep but the solving of this problem is really a matter for your family doctor, and if he or she thinks it necessary, for a skin specialist also.

## Tooth-grinding

Tooth-grinding, or bruxism as it is termed, is quite common, particularly among children. The tooth-grinder performs munching movements for perhaps ten seconds at a time, that recur frequently during the night. In adults the movements are sometimes brought on by drugs, but generally are a persistence of a childhood habit that has not been lost. It causes concern to dentists who find the teeth more worn away than would be expected, and it can be disconcerting for a bed-partner, at least at first. It does not signify any serious trouble, and certainly requires no treatment.

## Head-banging and body-rocking

Rhythmic head-banging and body-rocking, like sleep-walking, are more dramatic than significant. Rhythmic activity is relaxing and comforting: mother rocks the baby, granny sits in her rocking chair, and gum-chewing remains popular. Infants, whether they be infant monkeys, chimpanzees or humans, will often squat on their haunches and rock their bodies to and fro when they are frightened and lonely. Others suck their thumbs. So one child when put to bed will suck his thumb, and another will rock to and fro. The rocking may be a side-to-side movement of the head, perhaps with humming, or it may involve getting on to hands and knees and banging the head on the pillows.

It is commonest at around eighteen months to two years of age after which time it usually diminishes in frequency, eventually to disappear with the passing of years. A few children come to do it not only when they are first put to bed but actually during their sleep. They may do it recurrently during the middle of the night, so that the whole cot shakes violently. This is alarming to the parents, but in our experience, and to the best of our knowledge, no one –

child or adult – has come to any harm in this way.

Rarely, these movements persist into adult life, and there is nothing more remarkable than to see a large man asleep but hurling himself with extraordinary vigour from side to side, perhaps 100 times a minute and for as long as a minute, repeating the performance several times before the night is out.

Like sleep-walking, body-rocking at night does not signify any serious psychological abnormality, although episodes of body-rocking do occur more frequently at times when daytime anxiety is higher. It may be that the rocking is some kind of long-established comfort habit that is triggered off by an anxious mental episode during dreaming. Whatever the cause, once again, the passage of time usually sees the habit disappear.

# Night wanderings of the elderly

We all grow old, but we grow old at different rates. Some people retain complete lucidity of mind when they are ninety, while others are less favoured and their minds show the changes of old age when they are only seventy. When the ageing process in the brain is very rapid or far advanced, the brain's powers of organizing information and of forming new memories, so that tomorrow the events of today will easily be recalled, are much diminished. Under these circumstances sleep is greatly fragmented. There is relatively little paradoxical sleep, there is no deep orthodox sleep, and the night may be punctuated by clambering out of bed and wandering around the house or down the street in a confused state of wakefulness, with diminished awareness of surroundings and even lack of recognition of familiar faces. This kind of nocturnal wandering is common among the very elderly.

Getting lost can be bad enough by day, but things are much worse by night, without the stabilizing influences of ordinary daytime routines and of well-lit rooms. And to compound the difficulties, our biological clock, which helps us to be efficient by day, makes all of us less mentally efficient in the middle of the night. When this loss of efficiency comes on top of the impairments of old age, fairly severe mental confusion is especially likely in the night. If one of your family is prone to such episodes, then it is certainly worth taking the simple precautions we described in Chapter 4 for avoiding injury to sleep-walkers, and maybe even following the example we mentioned of the lawyer who used to hide his door key to prevent his sleep-walking taking him too far afield.

The nocturnal confusion and wanderings often come during the course of a mild chest or kidney infection and tend to arise more easily in unfamiliar surroundings, so that they often accompany a stay in hospital. Here, at least, the elderly are in the hands of staff trained to cope with just this sort of event.

Great caution has to be exercised in the use of drugs to help sleep for these older people, indeed many of the conventional sleeping pills, such as the barbiturates, only make matters worse. It requires guidance from an experienced medical adviser.

# Sleeping too much

Complaints about sleeping too much are less common than complaints of sleeping too little, and, to be precise, what is generally complained of is sleeping at inappropriate times. In the first chapter we noted that there are substantial individual differences in the amount of sleep people need. Some are perfectly happy and healthy with only three hours of sleep a night, most of us like seven or eight hours, and there are others who need ten or twelve. Given the chance there are a few people who will sleep for twenty-two hours in the twenty-four, though it is not something they can keep up day after day. If it is your natural pattern to have longer-than-average sleep you will probably find you have difficulty in getting up in the morning and take more sleep by day by having naps.

Those who have particular difficulty in waking up properly in the morning may suffer from what is termed 'sleep-drunkenness'. It is possible that they really need longer asleep, but it is more likely that their biological clock runs in such a way that full awakening is delayed. They tend to be confused and irritable when first awakened, and are often late for work. An afternoon or evening shift job may be the answer.

Sleeping too much is not always a matter of spending long hours in bed. There are three little-known conditions in which the sufferers fall asleep involuntarily during the day. They are: idiopathic narcolepsy, hypersomnia and sleep apnoea. We have already dealt with sleep apnoea in Chapter 6, since it is also a cause of insomnia at night.

### Idiopathic narcolepsy
This is a condition that affects around one person in a thousand, that

is to say some 50,000 in Britain alone. It can be a real nuisance for the sufferer, embarrassing, annoying and can have consequences that certainly need to be more widely understood.

Sufferers fall asleep once, twice or three times a day, for periods of about ten minutes, at times when they don't want to. Usually after a year or two of this, they also become subject to what are known as cataplectic attacks. These involve a brief loss of muscle strength for a period of a few seconds, affecting the whole or part of the body, and are triggered off by sudden emotion. In one person it is momentary anger that is responsible; in another, fear; in another, laughter; in yet another, triumph. The sleep attacks and the cataplectic attacks can come on at any age, though they usually do so in the earlier decades of life. In a few people they seem to go away in old age.

When most of us fall asleep we go into orthodox sleep and never immediately into paradoxical sleep, but the person with idiopathic narcolepsy quite often goes directly from wakefulness into paradoxical sleep. The cataplectic attack is in fact a half-hearted entry into paradoxical sleep, with the paralysis of the muscles, but only for a few seconds.

A common experience of the same phenomenon is sleep paralysis. Any of us can have a bad dream and, waking from paradoxical sleep, momentarily find ourselves paralyzed. The narcoleptic is particularly liable to be aware of episodes of sleep paralysis, not just at night, but at any time when he takes a sleep. Owing to their association with paradoxical sleep, vivid dreams – sometimes taking the form of nightmares – are particularly often remembered on waking from these involuntary daytime naps.

While any of us may on occasion fall asleep when we are bored on a bus or train, the narcoleptic falls asleep far more often in these situations so that he misses his stop. Engaged in work of a repetitive nature, he wakens to find that he has failed to attend to his duties for some minutes. The secretary wakes to find herself slumped across her typewriter, and discovers that she has typed nonsense for the last few lines before dropping off. Walking along the street, the young man becomes sleepier and sleepier, sees double, and is taken for drunk by passers-by. On another occasion he is playing table-tennis and is about to make a triumphant smash, when the muscles of his body suddenly go limp. The young mother has to sit down before her friends tell a joke, in case she laughs and drops the baby.

It is, of course, dangerous to drive or operate heavy machinery if you are a narcoleptic; hardly surprisingly, people with the condition have a high rate of accidents, often through running into the back of other vehicles.

Narcolepsy can strike at awkward times. A girl-friend, taken out to the cinema, will not think it complimentary when her young man quickly falls asleep beside her. The wife who has patiently prepared a good meal feels no encouragement if her husband then falls asleep in the middle of eating it. Among the most important things you can do as a sufferer is to try to help those close to you, and people at work, to understand that falling asleep is not a sign of sloth or lack of interest in their company, but is as much a disability as a peptic ulcer.

**Treatment** The cataplectic attacks are usually much less of a nuisance than the sleep episodes, though it is the sleep episodes that are the more difficult to treat. There are modern drugs, particularly one of the antidepressants called clomipramine (Anafranil), that very effectively get rid of the cataplectic attacks, while leaving the sleep trouble much the same.

There are other drugs that will reduce the frequency of sleep attacks and doctors vary in their attitudes to their use. We think it more important that you should avoid drugs and try to regulate the pattern of life so that the sleep attacks cause the least disturbance. If a deliberate nap is taken at the morning coffee-break, for example, and another opportunity to lie down is taken in the lunch hour, and yet another at the afternoon tea-break, then the involuntary naps are less likely to arise at awkward times.

### Hypersomnia

Hypersomnia affects about the same number of people as idiopathic narcolepsy – around one person in a thousand. Hypersomniacs differ from narcoleptics in that they do not have the hallmark of going direct into paradoxical sleep, and when they do fall asleep it is more often for half an hour to an hour at a stretch, perhaps three or four times per week. Again, their disability makes it dangerous for them to drive. Occasionally the time of onset can be traced back to an infectious illness or a head injury, but generally there is no identifiable cause.

**What can be done** Although there is no specific treatment for the condition, there are certain common-sense measures that can be taken. Obesity should be reduced, weight being brought down, if possible, to slightly under the ideal weight for height (see table on page 94); caffeine in pill form or from coffee may be used to help sustain alertness on important occasions; and once again it is most important that the family and colleagues at work should understand that the falling asleep does not represent laziness, unsociableness or lack of appreciation of their company.

# 10. GOLDEN RULES FOR BETTER SLEEP

We hope the preceding chapters have answered most of your questions about sleep. If they have also dispelled some of the misconceptions you had – have helped to sort out in your mind the fact from the fiction – and have allayed your worst fears about what bad sleep can mean for you, then the book will have achieved its purpose.

In this short concluding chapter we would like to set out our guidelines for better sleep. In effect, they sum up all we have said so far, and are intended also to provide a quick and easy source of reference for the future.

● Regular hours for getting up and going to bed will give you better sleep by night and more vigour by day.

● Regular early rising helps to ensure that you regularly fall asleep early.

● Remember that visions, voices and bodily jerks are the normal events of falling asleep.

● Although our bodies work very differently in orthodox and paradoxical sleep, we cannot influence how much of which kind of sleep we get. The brain will look after its own needs without our help.

● Don't give any credence to the mistaken belief that if you don't dream, you will go out of your mind. We all dream every night, though mostly we forget our dreams on waking.

● Don't be overanxious about your child if he has night-terrors or nightmares or sleep-walks. He can be expected to grow out of it fairly soon; he will remember nothing of these events in the morning; and it is only you who are distressed. If there are obvious daytime sources of worry, then even if they cannot be resolved immediately, they are probably going to right themselves with time.

If *you* have bad dreams or sleep-walk, think of alcohol or drugs as a possible cause. Whether for child or adult, simple precautions against injury are worth taking.

● If you have lost sleep, be reassured by the fact that sleep is an excellent self-regulating system. You will get sleep if you really need it.

● If you do not get as much sleep as you would like, the consequences will be less serious than your worst fears. However, you may be more irritable than usual, and so may your partner or close family when they are tired, too. To avoid making matters worse we all have to try and be relaxed and tolerant with each other, and to make allowances for the ill-temper bad sleep can cause.

● Monotony, warmth and satisfaction of basic needs tend to send us off to sleep quicker than their opposites.

● For better sleep and your general health and well-being, take plenty of regular daytime exercise. But if you are taking up an activity for the first time, take it easy to begin with.

● Before buying expensive luxury items for your home, think first whether the money could be better spent on a new bed. If you are sleeping badly on an old 'sagger', a bed with a firm sprung base and mattress is definitely a worthwhile investment.

● If you smoke and your sleep is bad, give up smoking; and whether you smoke or not, don't drink coffee, tea or cola drinks late in the evening.

● Never take slimming pills.

● Never use alcohol to get you to sleep.

● If your family doctor agrees that you should use sleeping pills to help you get back into what you feel is a natural pattern of sleep after a crisis in your life, try not to take them for more than two or three nights successively. The more modern benzodiazepines (see page 90) are the pills of choice in these circumstances. The best are those that do not build up in the body with repeated intake.

● Avoid being underweight or severely overweight. And if you are

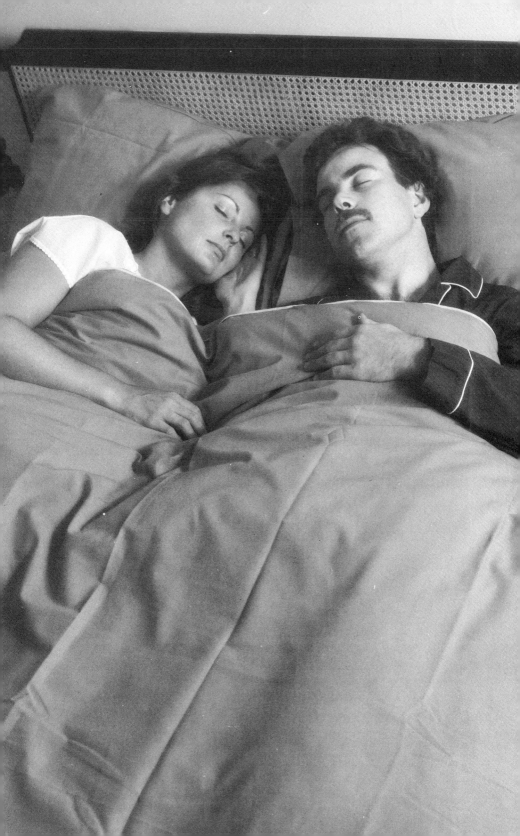

on or somewhat above your ideal weight, consider, before commencing a weight-reducing diet, which is more important to you: good sleep or a fashionable figure. For when you lose weight you will probably lose sleep also. Being a little on the chubby side does no harm, and in fact you may feel happier and sleep better like this than if you are leaner.

● Take your meals at regular times, not supper early one day and late the next. If you are accustomed to eat in the evening, let it be food that is easily digestible. Proprietary malted food drinks fall into this category, and do seem to be effective in promoting good sleep.

● Finally, be satisfied with yourself as you are, accepting your failures in life, your minor disabilities and that you perhaps feel you do not sleep as much as you would like.

We realize that to urge you to throw off your worries and the problems of life is a counsel of perfection, but we at least would like to feel that through this book we may have relieved some of your worries about sleep itself and that as a result you will indeed get a better night's sleep

# ACKNOWLEDGEMENTS

The publishers are grateful to the following individuals and organizations for their help in the preparation of this book.

For permission to reproduce photographs: AGE Fotostock, Barcelona (page 85); Colour Library International, London (page 56); the Goethe Museum, Frankfurt (page 44); Gruner & Jahr, Munich (page 68); Lufthansa (page 67); NFB Photothèque, Ottawa (page 15); the Photographers' Library, London (pages 25 and 52); and the Tate Gallery, London (page 37).

The cover and location photographs were taken by Dave Brown and Dave Robinson. Most of the modelling was done by Miriam Brewster, Richard Smith, and Jane and Peter Murray Hill. The bed and headboard were kindly lent by the London Bedding Centre, London, SW1; the bedwear by Dorma, London; the china and glass by the Reject Shop, King's Road, London; and the enuresis alarm by Wessex Medical Equipment Co Ltd, Romsey, Hampshire.

The diagrams on pages 11, 15, 21, 23, 26, 34, 35, 58, 73 and 88 were drawn by David Gifford. The reference for the diagram on page 58 is by courtesy of the London Bedding Centre.

Finally, thanks are due to Jennifer Eaton, BSc, MSc, MPS, for information on international drug name equivalents.

# APPENDIX: DRUG NAME EQUIVALENTS

| Approved name | UK Trade name | USA Trade name |
|---|---|---|
| amitriptyline | Tryptizol; Elavil | Elavil; Endep; SK-Amitriptyline; Amitid |
| amylobarbitone sodium / amobarbital sodium | Sodium Amytal | Amytal Sodium |
| barbitone / barbital | Veronal (no longer available) | not available |
| butobarbitone / butethal | Soneryl | not available |
| chloral hydrate | Noctec; Triclofos | Noctec; SK-Schloral Hydrate; Triclos |
| chlordiazepoxide | Librium | Librium; A-Poxide; SK-Lygen |
| clomipramine | Anafranil | not available |
| dexamphetamine / dextroamphetamine | Dexedrine | Dexedrine |
| diazepam | Valium | Valium |
| dichloralphenazone | Welldorm | available only as an ingredient of Midrin |
| flurazepam | Dalmane | Dalmane |
| glutethimide | Doriden | Doriden |
| imipramine | Berkomine; Tofranil | Tofranil; Janimine; SK-Pramine |
| lormetazepam | Noctamid | not yet available |
| meprobamate | Equanil | Equanil; Miltown; SK-Bamate |
| methaqualone + diphenhydramine | Mandrax (no longer available) | not available |
| nitrazepam | Mogadon | not available |
| paraldehyde | no trade name | no trade name |
| pentobarbitone sodium / pentobarbital sodium | Nembutal | Nembutal Sodium |
| phenmetrazine | Preludin (no longer available) | Preludin |
| phenobarbitone / phenobarbital | Luminal | Luminal; Solfoton; SK-Phenobarbital |
| potassium bromide | no trade name | no trade name |
| triazolam | Halcion | not available |
| tryptophan | Optimax; Pacitron | Trofan; Tryptacin |
| viloxazine | Vivalan | not available |

| Approved name | CANADA Trade name | AUSTRALIA Trade name | SOUTH AFRICA Trade name |
|---|---|---|---|
| amitriptyline | Elavil; Deprex; Levate, Meravil; Novotriptyn | Tryptanol; Elavil; Saroten; Laroxyl | Tryptanol; Saroten; Deprestat; Trepiline |
| amylobarbitone sodium } amobarbital sodium } | Sodium Amytal | Amytal Sodium; Amylobeta; Neur-Amyl Sodium | Amytal Sodium |
| barbitone } barbital } | not available | not available | not available |
| butobarbitone } butethal } | Soneryl | Soneryl; Sonabarb | Soneryl |
| chloral hydrate | Noctec; Chloralvan; Novochlorhydrate | Chloradorm; Dormel; Chloralix | Triclyoryl |
| chlordiazepoxide | Corax; Medilium; Librium; Relaxil | Librium | Librium; Chlortran |
| clomipramine | Anafranil | not available | Anafranil |
| dexamphetamine } dextroamphetamine } | Dexedrine | Sigma; Dexamphetamine | not available |
| diazepam | Valium; Meval; Rival; Vivol | Lorinon; Valium; Ducene; Pro-Pam | Valium; Betapam; Diatran; Nortense |
| dichloralphenazone | Choralol | Bonadorm | not available |
| flurazepam | Dalmane | Dalmane | Dalmadorm |
| glutethimide | Doriden | Doriden | not available |
| imipramine | Tofranil; Impril; Novopramine | Tofranil; Imiprin; Iramil; Melipramine | Tofranil |
| lormetazepam | not yet available | not yet available | Noctamid |
| meprobamate | Equanil; Miltown; Meditran; Quietal | Equanil; Mepron | Equanil; Meposed; Pantranquil |
| methaqualone + } diphenhydramine } | Mandrax | Mandrax | not available |
| nitrazepam | Mogadon | Mogadon; Dormicum | Mogadon; Hypnotin; Noctene; Ormodon |
| paraldehyde | no trade name | no trade name | no trade name |
| pentobarbitone sodium } pentobarbital sodium } | Nembutal; Pentogen | Nembutal; Pentone; Penbon | Nembutal |
| phenmetrazine | not available | not available | not available |
| phenobarbitone } phenobarbital } | Gardenal; Luminal; Nova-Pheno | available only as an ingredient in combination products | Gardenal |
| potassium bromide | no trade name | no trade name | no trade name |
| triazolam | Halcion | not available | Halcion |
| tryptophan | not available | not available | not available |
| viloxazine | not available | not available | not available |

# INDEX

46; spindles, 32
breathing difficulties, 70–1, 93
*British Medical Journal*, 91
bromides, 79, 80
bronchitis, 70
bruxism, 105

caffeine, 67, 76–7, 78, 110
cataleptic attacks, 108–9
cheese, as cause of nightmares, 44–5
chest disease, 70
children, apnoea, 70–1; bedwetting, 101–4; disturbed nights, 48, 50; growth hormones, 24; insomnia, 63; night-terrors, 43, 111–12; rhythmic movements, 104–6; sleep-walking, 42–3, 45–6, 111–12; threadworms, 69
chloral hydrate, 79–80, 82
chlordiazepoxide, 81–2, 86
cholecystokinin, 95–6
cigarette smoking, 75–6, 78, 112
circadian rhythm, 10–15, 26–7, 48
clomipramine, 109
cocoa, 77
coffee, 76–7, 78, 110, 112
cola drinks, 77, 112
corticosteroids, 22, 24, 26–7, 73–4
Crisp, Prof Arthur, 91, 92–3

Dalmane, 82, 83, 84, 86–7, 88, 90
day-dreaming, 18, 41
Dement, Dr, 38–9, 40–1
depression, antidepressant

drugs, 41, 66, 77, 102, 109; as cause of sleep-loss, 64–6
dexamphetamine, 77, 81, 102
Dexedrine, 102
diazepam, 82, 90
dieting, 77, 92–5, 114
diphenhydramine, 81
disease, and sleep-loss, 67–9, 70–1
diuretics, 77–8
doctors, sleep-loss, 50, 51
Doriden, 81
double beds, 58, 59
double-glazing, 67
dreams, 37–45, 111; bad dreams, 42–5; function of, 39–40, 41; lack of, 40–1; and types of sleep, 33; withdrawal from sleeping drugs, 88
Drexel, Dr, 98
drinks, bedtime, 98–100, 114
driving, as cause of sleepiness, 16
drowsiness, 18–19, 32
drugs, antidepressants, 41, 66, 77, 102, 109; for narcolepsy, 109; pain-killers, 67–9, 77; to prevent bed-wetting, 102; and sleep-walking, 46; stimulants, 75–8; *see also* sleeping drugs

ear-plugs, 67, 72
Elavil, 102
elderly, night wandering, 106–7; sleep loss, 62–3
electroencephalograph (EEG), 31–3, 43
enuresis, 101–4

*Other books in the*
*Positive Health Guide*
Series ✖

## HIGH BLOOD PRESSURE
*What it means for you, and how to*
*control it*
**Dr Eoin O'Brien and Professor Kevin**
**O'Malley**

Written by two eminent physicians, this is a comprehensive and
practical guide to detecting, preventing and controlling high blood
pressure – one of the most serious risks to health and life
expectancy. Special features include: illustrated step-by-step
instructions for measuring your own blood pressure, with
recommendations on the most suitable equipment to buy; a
detailed analysis of the factors that cause high blood pressure;
suggestions for getting exercise into your daily routine; and up-to-
date informtion on the action and side-effects of all the main
blood-pressure-lowering drugs in use today.

## ASTHMA & HAYFEVER
*How to relieve wheezing and sneezing*
**Dr Allan Knight**

A specialist in allergies and breathing difficulties shows how you
can cope with either of these common long-term problems. He
suggests practical ways to adjust your daily life to minimize
possible irritation to a sensitive nose or lungs. A special section has
been included to help children prone to asthmatic coughing and
wheezing. And several easy exercises are described to help you
relax and overcome the problem.

# THE HIGH-FIBRE COOKBOOK
*Recipies for good health*
**Pamela Westland**
**Introduced by Dr Denis Burkitt**

Here at last is a book that combines the healthy benefits of high-fibre eating with good imaginative home cooking. Bestselling cookery writer Pamela Westland presents over 200 delicious tried-and-tested high-fibre recipes for all occasions, backed up with plenty of helpful advice on preparing this kind of food, as well as unusual and appetizing serving suggestions. As a useful slimmers' guide, each recipe is accompanied by its fibre, calorie and fat values; and over seventy are illustrated in superb colour photographs.

# THE DIABETICS' DIET BOOK
*A new high-fibre eating programme*
**Dr Jim Mann and the Oxford Dietetic Group**

The first book for diabetics and their dieticians that shows how to change to the new high-carbohydrate-and-fibre diet now being recommended by leading diabetic organizations around the world.

Well-known diabetologist Dr Jim Mann and his experienced team explain how easy it is to change to this approach, and how it will improve diabetic control.

They present over 140 delicious and carefully tested recipes that will appeal to diabetics and their families as well. All the dishes are accompanied by a comprehensive nutritional analysis and many have been temptingly brought to life in sixteen pages of specially taken colour photographs.